International Perspectives
on State and Family Support
for the Elderly

International Perspectives on State and Family Support for the Elderly

Scott A. Bass, PhD
Robert Morris, DSW
Editors

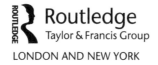

Routledge
Taylor & Francis Group

LONDON AND NEW YORK

First published 1993 by The Haworth Press, Inc.

Published 2013 by Routledge
2 Park Square, Milton Park, Abingdon, Oxfordshire OX14 4RN
711 Third Avenue, New York, NY 10017, USA

First issued in paperback 2016

Routledge is an imprint of the Taylor & Francis Group, an informa business

International Perspectives on State and Family Support for the Elderly has also been published as *Journal of Aging & Social Policy*, Volume 5, Numbers 1/2 1993.

Library of Congress Cataloging-in-Publication Data

International perspectives on state and family support for the elderly / Scott A. Bass, Robert Morris, editors.
     p. cm.
    "Has also been published as Journal of aging & social policy, volume 5, numbers 1/2 1993"– T. p. verso.
    Includes bibliographical references (p.   ) and index.
    1. Aged-Government policy–Cross-cultural studies. 2. Aged-Care–Government policy–Cross-cultural studies. I. Bass, Scott A. II. Morris, Robert, 1910- .
HV1451.I548 1993
362.6–dc20   93-32907
                                                    CIP

ISBN 13: 978-1-138-97308-4 (pbk)
ISBN 13: 978-1-56024-480-6 (hbk)

International Perspectives on State and Family Support for the Elderly

CONTENTS

ABOUT THE EDITORS

Scott A. Bass, PhD, is Director of the Gerontology Institute at the University of Massachusetts at Boston and also Director of the University's PhD Program in Gerontology. He is co-editor of *Achieving a Productive Aging Society* (1993), *Diversity in Aging* (1989), and *Retirement Reconsidered* (1988) as well as co-editor of the *Journal of Aging & Social Policy*.

Robert Morris, DSW, Kirstein Professor Emeritus, Brandeis University, is a Senior Fellow at the Gerontology Institute, University of Massachusetts at Boston, and the University's Cardinal Meideros Visiting Lecturer. He is co-editor of *Retirement Reconsidered* and of the *Journal of Aging & Social Policy.*

Foreword:
"De-Constructing" Family Care Policy
for the Elderly:
A Note

John McCallum, DPhil

The Australian National University,
Canberra

In November 1991, while reviewing a program creating awareness of aging in Indonesia, Malaysia, Philippines, Singapore, and Thailand (McCallum & Osteria, 1992), I was consistently told that family support remained effective in the provision of welfare for the elderly despite increasing family mobility. This story was consistent across countries, service agencies, government departments, and even international agencies served by expatriates. However, outside these official and predominately male groups, this idealized view of family support for the aged did not hold true. One case can serve to illustrate this.

A senior woman academic from one of the countries reported to me an incident that had received considerable press coverage. In a fast-growing fringe settlement providing wage laborers for new

John McCallum, who has been International View editor of the *Journal of Aging & Social Policy* for the past three years, is Senior Research Fellow at the National Centre for Epidemiology and Population Health at the Australian National University, Canberra.

[Haworth co-indexing entry note]: Foreword: " 'De-Constructing' Family Care Policy for the Elderly: A Note," McCallum, John. Co-published simultaneously in the *Journal of Aging & Social Policy*, (The Haworth Press, Inc.) Vol. 5, No. 1/2, 1993, pp. 1-5; and: *International Perspectives on State and Family Support for the Elderly* (ed: Scott A. Bass and Robert Morris) The Haworth Press, Inc., 1993, pp. 1-5. Multiple copies of this article/chapter may be purchased from The Haworth Document Delivery Center [1-800-3-HAWORTH; 9:00 a.m. - 5:00 p.m. (EST)].

1

urban industries, a majority of families were placing their elderly early each day, sometimes with little sustenance, in an open field without shade and collecting them in the evening. The pressures of work and getting children to education had left no time for traditional family care. There was no day care and they could not have afforded it even if it had been available. The media reports headlined the shameful nature of the situation but also stressed the decline in the ability of families to provide support.

In the view of my expert informer, it was clearly the case that the traditional family support system often could not provide adequate care of the elderly in the industrializing areas of rapidly developing Asian countries. However, policymakers were unable to see the need for public or at least community support for families with elderly members. It was not simply that they were unable to provide it, they did not perceive that there was a need for it. Was it because they were mostly men and insensitive to the burdens of care, or perhaps because they were public officials wishing to present their society in a positive light? How could they have neglected such public cases when they were apparently reporting honestly to me the continued viability of traditional family support? A similar situation had arisen in earlier times in developed countries like Great Britain (Laslett, 1989) and a current investigation of family care in 16 countries (Kosberg, 1992, p. 298) has concluded that "many countries reflect an apprehension that the provision of alternatives to family care may be seen to legitimize and encourage the abandonment of family caregiving responsibilities."

This gap between official and lived reality is a key to the nature of family support policy development. Economic and demographic changes provide an imperative for new policy development but the social construction of the debates gives essential form to these developments. The specifics of this organized social activity vary between countries with different institutional structures, different levels of economic development, and with varying cultural values but the process is consistently influential.

Despite this, the demographic and economic imperatives influencing family support policies for the elderly usually attract greater attention than the social construction of the terms of policy debates. Because the support of close, intimate relations is so central to the satisfactory conduct of everyday life, "family" and "care" are vigorously contested terms everywhere. People are often unwilling and unable to deal with such central values in public debate. Even when they do, it is difficult to express deep but unconsciously held values and to bring such debates to satisfactory resolution. The policy contexts for increasing support to families caring for the elderly are perhaps less dramatic in other more developed countries but they can be equally conflictual as those in rapidly developing countries. Social construction of these debates occurs primarily through definitions and values that determine types of argument.

The definition of "family" is complex, with multiple types as well as considerable variation within types. The concepts of "extended families," "stem families," "modified extended families" and so on attempt to capture the rich variety of the primary groups to which individuals belong. Even when these forms can be clearly defined, they work differently when they are set within different institutional structures, different levels of economic development, and varying cultural values. As these settings change through time, the lived reality of family also changes. Because of this complexity alone, there is a need to examine critically concepts and definitions of "family" within any debate in which they are central terms.

"Family" is also a highly politicized term. So along with definitional complexity there are polarized or multiple readings of what is going on at any time in families. Men see things differently from women, heterosexuals from homosexuals, public officials from family caregivers, and traditionalists will read the current information about families differently from libertarians.

Family is classic territory for the creation of perceptions of "social problems" that require public intervention. Because of their capacity to draw on primary emotional responses, family issues can also be used to mask less popular political agendas. Cuts to family support can be dressed up positively as a return to the family supporting its own members. People with different ideological backgrounds will also differ as to whether or not they think that they have had "the wool pulled over their eyes" in particular cases of support.

The reality of "caregiving" is equally complex. This is easiest to see at the micro level in multidirectional, multiple-type flows between individuals within networks. These are influenced by equally intricate institutional and political structures, particularly within federated states. In population surveys, the constraints on what is defined as "caregiving" that are encountered when survey questions are constructed filter the picture of what is happening in caregiving.

When the Australian Bureau of Statistics (1990) defined caregiving as assistance provided by the major caregiver who co-resides with severely handicapped persons–using a World Health Organization-type definition–it produced a picture of caregiving as primarily a spousal activity, and a generational solidarity, in which men were equally as likely to provide care as women, even at older ages. This definition was congruent with the definitions used by the Department of Social Security for the payment of Carers Benefits. Less restrictive definitions of caregiving from other countries, particularly those including nonresident caregivers, show more intergenerational support along with generational solidarity and a greater prevalence of women as caregivers. However, it would be a mistake to regard any survey as providing the definitive view of caregiving. There are different ways of cutting up the complex and various perspectives on the multiplex flows that constitute caregiving.

The "social construction" of the terms and debates about family and caregiving to the elderly dictates a need for critical analysis in any discussion. "De-construction" here is the task of analyzing and understanding the powerful social and political forces that construct the political agendas for the public support of family caregiving to the elderly. This task is more obviously needed, and more crucial, when comparative study of different societies is involved. The diversity of values and institutions between societies can make the commonality of terms illusory relative to actual social forms.

The contributions in this collection, which respond to this task, provide a fresh range of lucid, sometimes comparative, analyses of family caregiving policy. Among the issues discussed are: the rights of caregivers and the potential for shifting burdens of care to private families in Canada, a review of policies for paying caregivers in Europe and the United States, the importance of family care in Sweden where public support is the most extensive and a comparison to Israel, the effects of frameworks of federalism in the United States and Canada, the Austrian preference for providing services rather than cash payments to caregivers, the range of policies that effect the well-being of caregivers in Canada, the impact of political agenda on care in China, and the changes in support in Denmark and Hong Kong along with the re-orientation to welfare pluralism in Great Britain. These are all important contributions to the task of analyzing and understanding policies for family caregiving. The papers and the debates themselves need to be read critically. It befits the most important but least visible area of policy for the aged that it should be debated vigorously and publicly deconstructed.

REFERENCES

Australian Bureau of Statistics. (1990). *Carers of the handicapped at home.* Canberra: ABS Cat.No.4112.0.

Kosberg, J.I. (1992). *Family care of the elderly: Social and cultural changes.* Newbury Park, CA: Sage Publications.

Laslett, P. (1989). *A fresh map of life: The emergence of the third age.* London: Weidenfeld and Nicolson.

McCallum, J., & Osteria T. (1992). *Creation of awareness on aging for policy making purposes in the Asian region.* Tokyo: Japanese Organization for International Cooperation in Family Planning Inc.

Introduction:
A Global View of Changing State and Family Support for Older Persons

Charlotte Nusberg

International Federation on Ageing
AARP International Information Center on Aging

From my perch as editor of an international journal looking at aging policies and programs and as Secretary-General of the International Federation on Ageing (IFA) for the past three years, I have witnessed some remarkable changes in state support for the elderly around the world. Many are double-edged, promising enhanced benefit while creating significant risk. Their evolution is being monitored closely by organizations representing or serving the aging–those organizations constituting the membership of the IFA.

These changes have been introduced largely in response to demographic and political pressures, ideological imperatives, economic constraints, and the promising results of social experimentation. Relatively few of these changes were initiated as a result of grass-roots demand–from older persons themselves or from any other

Charlotte Nusberg is Secretary-General of the International Federation on Ageing, Editor of *Ageing International,* and Director of AARP's International Information Center on Aging.

[Haworth co-indexing entry note]: Introduction: "A Global View of Changing State and Family Support for Older Persons," Nusberg, Charlotte. Co-published simultaneously in the *Journal of Aging & Social Policy,* (The Haworth Press, Inc.) Vol. 5, No. 1/2, 1993, pp. 7-11; and: *International Perspectives on State and Family Support for the Elderly* (ed: Scott A. Bass and Robert Morris) The Haworth Press, Inc., 1993, pp. 7-11. Multiple copies of this article/chapter may be purchased from The Haworth Document Delivery Center [1-800-3-HAWORTH; 9:00 a.m. - 5:00 p.m. (EST)].

significant political constituency. Nor has the so-called generational "backlash" that is sometimes read about in the press been influential in this process.

INCOME ADEQUACY

By and large, the income position of today's elderly in the more developed countries has not deteriorated over the last decade despite global recession and real income losses on the part of some younger age groups. In some cases, for example, France and Ireland, it has even improved. This has not been true of many developing countries where older people have experienced sharp declines in their living standards along with most of the rest of the population. There may, in fact, be fewer older persons protected by social security systems in developing countries–for example, in Latin America–than was the case in the 1970s.

Several industrialized countries–for example, the United Kingdom, Austria, Denmark, and Australia–have moved in the direction of privatizing their publicly supported pension systems and/or placing greater reliance on occupational pensions as a major source of retirement income. And several developing countries–Chile is a prime example–have gone so far as to privatize their entire pension system. Further, the Chilean model is being examined with great interest by the newly liberated societies of Eastern Europe, which see in it great potential for relieving the public purse in the years ahead. The debate over who is to assume responsibility for income security protection in old age is, in fact, becoming quite heated.

The potential for public savings over time as population aging continues was, of course, a key motivation behind the movement to privatize pensions. It is not at all clear, however, that savings will result–much less that tomorrow's elderly will be protected. Much hinges on the wisdom of individuals in choosing appropriate pension funds and of pension fund managers in making sound investments. In case of failure or default, will the public sector be able to serve as the protector of last resort? Are governments even planning for such a contingency? What about the large majority of the population in most developing nations that remains outside the formal sector and does not qualify to join a private plan? To whom will they turn? Will we see a reliance on means- or income-testing for obtaining public assistance?

Other important social security changes that have taken place in several countries are the raising of the age for pension eligibility–for example, the United States and Germany–and the tightening of conditions for early retirement. These, too, have been introduced to help stabilize social security financing. Such changes make sense at several levels. However, the impact of these changes on those persons who cannot find appropriate work or whose health militates against their continuing employment has not been well thought through.

The one major change in social security protection that may have had more of the interest of older persons at heart than macro-economic objectives is the gradual expansion of partial pensions throughout Scandinavia and parts of Western Europe. Partial pensions permit older persons to continue to work on a part-time basis while drawing a partial pension either before or after the normal pensionable age. As such, partial pensions hold open the promise of retirement "a la carte." To date, however, they do not seem to be very popular–either with employers or potential beneficiaries.

THE RETREAT FROM UNIVERSALISM

Parallel with efforts to privatize pension provision has been a retreat from universalist principles in several more developed countries towards a system of pluralist provision or a public/private mix of social services. This retreat has been particularly evident in the welfare states of the United Kingdom, the Netherlands, and, to a lesser extent, Sweden.

From a situation where the public sector was responsible for providing all those in need with appropriate social services, these countries have moved towards recognizing a pluralist system of service provision coordinated through a publicly supported case management process. The important roles that the family, the voluntary sector, and the commercial sector can play alongside the public sector in care provision are now recognized and encouraged.

The reforms were undertaken ostensibly to increase choice for the consumer and design a flexible package of services tailored to individual need–all, it is hoped, at lower cost to the public purse than the previous practice. The reforms may also have the effect of targeting public services on persons with the greatest need–that is, those very frail persons without financial resources and/or family support. If so, public services may again become a residual system for those persons who, because of a variety of life contingencies, have not been able to arrange for their well-being in old age. One danger of this is that the high quality of public services provided or at least sought under universal systems may deteriorate as they become targeted to the poor alone. Another possible effect of the reforms is that while they may provide more satisfactory care to some, they also may serve to increase inequality in old age. Universalist provision had the effect of leveling upward.

The role of the family becomes key in assuring appropriate care for frail older persons under these reforms. The reforms are admirable in that they formally recognize the important contributions family members are already making, but they also carry the threat of shifting the costs of care from the formal to the informal sector. Further, to what extent will family members welcome being "managed?" Can the act of management even threaten family care itself? Clearly, families can be either empowered or disempowered through the case management process, depending on how this function is carried out. The reforms are still too new to know how they will actually play out in practice.

FAMILY CARE IN DEVELOPING NATIONS

Ten years following the United Nations World Assembly on Aging there is at least a recognition on the part of policymakers in developing nations that families often need some outside support if they are to continue to carry out their traditional roles of caregiving for frail elders. Unfortunately, few have been able to follow through and enact the policies and programs to make that support a reality.

Yet the plight of elders is becoming more serious as the extended family continues to break down under the inexorable pressures of internal and external migration, urbanization, and modernization. Added to this are the new "grandparenting" responsibilities imposed upon elders in both developing and more developed nations as growing numbers of the middle generation are wiped out or rendered ineffective by AIDS or by drug or alcohol abuse.

CONCLUSION

Population aging is certainly serving as a catalyst for important policy changes. Whether all these changes will be beneficial remains to be seen. It will be critical for organizations that represent and serve the elderly to monitor carefully the impact of these changes and make recommendations for addressing the problems that do occur.

REFERENCES

Baldock, J., & Evers, A. (1991, June). Innovations and care of the elderly: The front line of change for social welfare services. *Ageing International, XVIII* (1), 8-21.

Hoskins, D., & Hoskins, I. (1992, December). The prospects for income security ten years later. *Ageing International, XIX* (4), 11-16.

GENERAL ARTICLES

The Effects of Federalism on Policies for Care of the Aged in Canada and the United States

Phoebe S. Liebig, PhD

University of Southern California, Los Angeles

SUMMARY. Debates about who should care for the elderly often center on the relative responsibilities of the state and family. In federal societies such as Canada and the United States, however, *multiple* governments are involved. This article compares and contrasts federalism in these two nations and its effects on the division of fiscal, administrative, and programmatic responsibilities for care of the aged between the national and regional (i.e., state, provincial) governments. Two major policy arenas, health care and social services,

Phoebe S. Liebig is Assistant Professor of Gerontology and Public Administration at the University of Southern California. She is the author of several journal articles and reports on state-level policy and on the effects of federalism on aging and aging-related policy in the United States and other nations.

[Haworth co-indexing entry note]: "The Effects of Federalism on Policies for Care of the Aged in Canada and the United States," Liebig, Phoebe S. Co-published simultaneously in the *Journal of Aging & Social Policy,* (The Haworth Press, Inc.) Vol. 5, No. 1/2, 1993, pp. 13-37; and: *International Perspectives on State and Family Support for the Elderly* (ed: Scott A. Bass and Robert Morris) The Haworth Press, Inc., 1993, pp. 13-37. Multiple copies of this article/chapter may be purchased from The Haworth Document Delivery Center [1-800-3-HAWORTH; 9:00 a.m. - 5:00 p.m. (EST)].

13

are examined, with particular attention focused on the roles played by the nongovernmental sector. Because most care of the aged is provided informally–a situation firmly rooted in the value systems and public policies of both nations–national and regional policies that assist family caregivers *directly* are examined. Policymakers at the regional level have been more active and often more innovative in constructing policies that are supportive of family caregiving, but in general, few programs of direct assistance exist in either nation and these largely depend on their geographic location. The article concludes with a discussion of the continued effects of federalism for future policies affecting care of the aged and suggests some approaches that can be undertaken to empower families in their care-giving roles.

Debates about who should care for the elderly often center on the relative responsibilities of the state and the family (Moroney, 1986). In federal societies such as Canada and the United States, however, *multiple* governments are involved. These two North American neighbors are linked by history, geography, and heritage, as well as comparably diverse populations with a similar distribution of living standards and shared concerns about care for the aged. Recent swings towards greater decentralization and devolution in both have been accompanied by national government grants with fewer strings attached, greater regional (provincial or state) government involvement in domestic affairs, and increased reliance on market strategies and the voluntary sector (Chandler & Bakvis, 1989; Pagano & Bowman, 1989). In this current policy climate, defining who should care for the elderly includes redefining responsibilities of national and regional governments.

This article presents an analysis of policies affecting the care of the aged in Canada and the United States, with a special focus on the framework of federalism and its effects on those policies. It first compares and contrasts national-regional government relationships in both nations by noting the value orientations about the role of government and the nature of intergovernmental relations. A second section describes the major divisions of fiscal, administrative, and programmatic responsibilities for care of the aged between the two levels of government in two major policy arenas: (1) health care and (2) social services. It also examines the extent to which these policies are age-neutral or age-specific, universal or income/means tested, and the roles played by the nongovernmental sector (i.e., voluntary, informal, commercial) in both nations.

Because most care of the aged is provided informally–a situation firmly rooted in the value systems and public policies of both nations (Chappell, 1990; Doty, 1986)–a third section focuses on national and regional policies that assist family caregivers *directly,* e.g., direct payment for services, promotion of corporate eldercare, family leave laws, respite care, and caregiver training and support. The article concludes with a brief discussion of the implications for the future of current Canadian and American trends in federalism, and their likely effects on determining who should care for the elderly.

THE FRAMEWORK OF FEDERALISM

Under federalism, a national government and one or more subnational levels of government each enjoy substantial policy-making powers and enter into arrangements for working out solutions, making joint decisions, and adopting joint policies (Nathan, 1990). A complex set of relationships results which can be described as independent (autonomous), interdependent (negotiated), or dependent (hierarchical). These relationships are also dynamic, with constant shifts and realignments blurring the boundaries of effective jurisdiction, resulting in the "marble cake federalism" that is characteristic of Canada and the United States (Burgess, 1990; Hanson, 1990). Some posit that the marble cake now has at least four "flavors," because of the increasing reliance on the nongovernmental sector and local governments (Bloksberg, 1989; Landes, 1983; Pagano & Bowman, 1989; Stevenson, 1985).

The federal system is often adopted in democratic nations, such as Canada and the United States, to ensure that governmental power is not concentrated; rather, it is fragmented among several levels. In addition, federal systems often serve to reconcile competing and conflicting diversities such as the accommodation of ethnic, linguistic, and institutional roots, as well as afford more points of access for the voicing of citizen preferences (Bowman & Pagano, 1990; Hanson, 1990; Wagenberg, Soderlund, Nelson, & Briggs, 1990; Watts, 1990).

Despite this basic agreement on the need for fragmented power, views about the legitimacy of government are different. Historically, there has been a strong mistrust of government in the United States. The nongovernmental sector is viewed as more capable of solving problems; government, at any level, should intervene only as a last resort (Borgatta & Montgomery, 1987; Linsk, Keigher, Simon-Rusinowitz, & England, 1992; Lipset, 1991). By contrast, the Canadian view towards government is mildly positive, with historic approval of government's use to achieve private ends and ensure social justice whether by public or nonpublic programs (Brink, 1992; Presthus, 1974). In Canada, regional governments (provinces) have enjoyed a fair measure of public approval, with the federal government often regarded more negatively (Presthus, 1974, p. 26); in the United States, the reverse has generally been true (Van Horn, 1989). This contrast may stem from greater clarity about the relative responsibilities of the two levels of government in Canada. Its constitution is far more explicit about the powers and authority of the provinces.

In the two nations, strong similarities occur in national-regional relationships in major areas of consequential powers (Nathan, 1990): the legal powers of regional polities to establish and revise their own political structures and processes, and over local governments; regional government responsibility for health and social services with concurrent national government involvement; and strong historical, social, and cultural identification of states and provinces, with their own political traditions of being more or less activist (Bickerton, 1990; Dye, 1990; Lammers & Klingman, 1984b; Leach, 1981). Major differences, however, are also evident in the ability of regional governments in the two nations to determine the kind and amounts of revenue they raise, how those revenues are to be shared by the national and regional polities, and their roles in shaping the affairs of the central government.

In the United States, states are able to levy taxes on a variety of sources, but with considerable variation among them (e.g., some have no state income tax); in most instances, the types of taxes raised by the national and state governments are the same. To promote national objectives, grants are provided to the states and local governments, and nonprofit and voluntary organizations, for health and social services. By contrast, provincial governments are precluded from levying taxes on major sources of revenue (e.g., broadbased consumption, income). Instead, based on negotiated agreements, the central government raises taxes on behalf of the regional governments and then shares the resulting revenue with them. Provincial governments retain powers to raise revenues; those that do not raise the average federal per capita tax receive equalization payments from the central government. Funding is provided to nonprofit/community groups for delivery of services to the elderly and others. In both nations, the regional governments want a bigger piece of the tax pie, largely because the recent emphasis on decentralization has left them with greater policy responsibilities than they can fund themselves (Bowman & Pagano, 1990; Burgess, 1990). They, in turn, are seeking to promote regional activities via participation of local authorities and the nongovernmental sector.

Even greater differences exist among the two nations in terms of the roles played by regional governments in central government affairs. Canada has eschewed formal representation of the 10 provinces in the upper house of national legislature. By contrast, the United States opted for equal representation of the 50 states, with Senators voting primarily for their individual state interests, rather than as a bloc representing state-level concerns.

The maintenance of national-regional relationships is also markedly different. In Canada, the principle of "executive federalism" undergirds a system of periodic conferences convened by federal and state executives and of negotiated agreements that require timely evaluation (Chandler & Bakvis, 1989). Intergovernmental task forces are also convened, often at the request of the provinces, to address major concerns such as long-term care. The parliamentary form of government and the relatively small numbers of regional governments promote this kind of exchange and bargaining. In the United States, however, few formal mechanisms exist for negotiating federal-state interactions, and there is a pattern of federal preemption extended to responsibilities that were previously acknowledged as state concerns (Zimmerman, 1991). The U.S. Advisory Commission on Intergovernmental Relations established by Congress largely acts as a source of information to federal and state policymakers, rather than as a broker. State officials have developed patterns of interstate consultation through formal associations (e.g., the National Governors Association, the National Conference of State Legislatures) that lobby at the national level, but they are but one of many public and private groups trying to gain the attention of Congress or the President. Thus, the nature of U.S. federalism is characterized by a mix of autonomous and hierarchical relations, in contrast to Canada's pattern of negotiated interdependence.

FEDERALISM AND HEALTH AND SOCIAL SERVICE POLICIES FOR THE AGED

The policy environment affecting the elderly in both nations is complex, given the involvement of several levels of government and the private sector in the policymaking, financing, and administration of health and social services. The current and projected numbers of older persons in Canada and the United States have, in part, led to central government efforts on their behalf, especially in the area of income security; concerns about their needs for other kinds of assistance; and the creation of special agencies: the Canadian Ministry of Health and Welfare for Seniors and the U.S. Administration on Aging. Responsibility for the aged is not either national government's alone; rather, it is shared with the regional governments and with the nongovernmental sector.

Health Policy for the Aged

As shown in Table 1, "Federalism and Health Services for the Aged in Canada and the United States," there are major differences between these nations in health policy affecting the elderly. The United States relies very heavily on the private sector for financing and increasingly on the national government for standard setting and regulation (Hanson, 1990; Zimmerman, 1990). The role of private insurance is a very major distinction, as is the lack of a national health plan, *except* for the elderly via Medicare that is financed by payroll taxes on employers and employees, by beneficiary premiums, and federal tax revenues. A national, means-tested health plan, Medicaid, exists for some (not all) of the poor, including the elderly poor, and is jointly financed by the national and state governments (although not equally so by all states). A large proportion of older Americans purchase private insurance ("Medigap") to supplement Medicare coverage; regulatory standards have been enacted at the national level and must be administered by the states in accordance with that legislation. Restrictions on Medicare payment levels for hospital and physician services have been passed, placing a greater burden on the aged and their families.

By contrast, Canada's federally and provincially financed health care system has universal coverage for conventional hospital and medical care, with all Canadians covered by the same plan. This program of medically necessary services is administered by the provinces; some receive equalization payments to ensure the same level of health services for all Canadians, *regardless of age*. Private insurers may not sell supplementary coverage for publicly insured services; doctors have essentially been prevented from charging patients anything above the government's fee schedule (Marmor, 1991).

Shared by the two nations, however, has been the emphasis on nursing home services as a major component of health care for the elderly and the setting of national standards for that care. (While nursing homes are also a housing arrangement–a fact recognized by Canadian policies requiring individuals to pay for the "pure" housing cost–most of what is provided is health care.) Joint national-regional government financing is the norm, although the proportions paid vary, as is the growing trend of providing community nursing or home health care, partly to restrain costs. The Medicaid program pays for more than 40% of nursing home care; waivers permit the delivery of noninstitutional care.

In Canada, regional governments play major roles in financing and administering health care, accompanied by national government co-financing and broad outlines for eligibility and administration. Acute and long-term care services are structured by the provinces through negotiated prices with hospitals, nursing homes, and physicians. A pattern of provincial autonomy results in significant variations in long-term care services and costs, similar to the United States. Six of the 10 provinces provide some insurance for nursing

Table 1.
FEDERALISM AND HEALTH SERVICES FOR THE AGED IN CANADA AND THE UNITED STATES

	CANADA	UNITED STATES
NATIONAL	Universal health insurance for medically necessary services Grants to provinces with equalization payments for poorer ones; set guidelines for provincial administration Capping of national support (38%) Extended Health Service Program doesn't cover nursing home care Little encouragement of nursing home construction Some funding for research Delivers services in territories, to veterans	National health insurance for aged, disabled - Medicare Health services for poor (including aged) - joint funding with states (50-83%) - Medicaid; requires states to expand coverage Sets standards for states to administer (nursing homes, "Medi-gap" insurance, assessment) Funding for research, training Delivery of services: veterans and native Americans
REGIONAL (PROVINCE/ STATE)	Administer universal health program Lot of variation in long-term care: nursing homes insured in 6; some cover drugs, eye glasses, personal care homes; home care not tied to physician approval Negotiate limits on hospital budgets, doctor fees; some with nursing homes; regulate nursing homes, provide grants to non-profit homes. Some moving toward payroll taxes to supplant premiums, some with user fees	Medicaid - joint funding; waivers permit flexibility for non-institutional care Own source revenues for health and mental health, drug assistance Some assessment programs Regulation of hospitals, nursing homes, private long-term care insurance, licensing of professionals Few fund research; more fund training; state hospitals Must pay Medicare premiums for poor aged.
LOCAL	Receive grants for hospital care Not big role in health area	Big delivery system, especially at the county level Zoning codes for health care facilities

FOR-PROFIT	Minor private insurance industry Providers negotiate with provinces about fees Important roles as owners of nursing homes, hospitals	Big role for private insurance industry; employers as source of retiree health. Private (for profit) hospitals, doctors, home nursing; 3/4 of nursing homes are proprietary Fee for service medicine (few controls) Big role of organizations of doctors, hospitals, and nursing homes
VOLUNTARY NON-PROFIT	Some nursing home ownership Receive provincial grants for long-term care patients and for charges to pay for operating deficits Important source of donations, services delivery, hospital ownership Health organizations receive federal grants to enhance seniors' health	Role of religious organizations and other voluntary groups; nursing homes, hospitals 20% of nursing homes are non-profit owned, operated Important source of donations, free time for services delivery
INDIVIDUAL, FAMILIES	Payment of premiums for coverage - those unable to pay, get assistance Permanent long-term care residents in hospitals may have to pay for meals	Pay Medicare premiums Purchase private insurance to supplement Medicare ("Medi-gap"), for out-of-pocket costs

21

home care, while four states have cosponsored the sale of such insurance, largely based on the incentives provided by a private foundation.

Regional government-funded home health services also show wide variations in both nations, for example, pharmaceutical assistance in the United States and coverage of personal care homes in Canada. In the former, however, the national government has enacted a number of Medicaid mandates that tend to reduce the states' flexibility in the use of the revenues they raise themselves (Lammers & Liebig, 1990), as does the requirement that the states must pay Medicare premiums for the poor elderly. While allowing states to use Medicaid funds for noninstitutional long-term care, the enactment of increasingly numerous national care standards sets up regulatory tensions between the two levels of government.

The two nations also share some similarities. The national government provides some health care services directly to veterans, indigenous populations, and persons residing in the territories. Local governments in the United States, however, play a much larger role in health care delivery, partly as an outgrowth of the 1960s and 1970s deinstitutionalization movement, which led to a marked decrease in the number of state hospitals and mental hospitals.

The roles of the commercial sector differ markedly. As noted earlier, the private insurance industry and employers play major roles in the United States. While nursing home fees are subject to specific reimbursement levels and at least a third or more of nursing homes are owned by the proprietary sector in both nations, Canada has a lower percentage of for-profit ownership. Provider associations play major roles in the setting or negotiation of fees and in political and lobbying activities in both Canada and the United States.

The roles of the voluntary sector in health care are also similar, both in the provision of institutional and home nursing services, although the proportions of ownership are generally smaller than those of the proprietary sector. In Canada, however, a pattern obtains of direct subsidies and grants to nonprofit groups including nursing homes and corporations run by community boards to deliver health and social services (NACA, 1990a). Subsidies to such organizations in the United States are usually provided indirectly via tax exemptions from all governmental levels.

Several patterns emerge regarding the ways in which responsibility for health services for the aged is apportioned among the public and private sectors in the two nations. The elderly have access to a national plan of acute health care, but their access to nursing home care and other long-term care services is largely determined at the regional level, usually guided by national government standards. In the United States, national health is available on either an age or means-tested basis; in Canada, far more is left to the regional governments which play major roles in the policymaking, financing, and administration of universal health care, based on federal-provincial and provincial-provider negotiations. Recent capping of federal support, however, may change this balance with provinces having to make forced choices. In the United States, federal-state interactions are characterized by a more hierarchical approach. In both nations, however, because certain health care issues are delegated, great variation occurs in health services for long-term care. Essentially, neither country has a national and universal long-term care policy.

The situation is further complicated by the federal-level provision of services to particular groups or geopolitical regions; by the heavy reliance on the voluntary sector which receives subsidies from one or more levels of government; and in the United States, by the health care roles played by local governments. The commercial sector is heavily engaged in the ownership and operation of nursing homes with regulatory restrictions imposed by the Canadian regional governments or by both levels in the United States. As a general rule, high levels of decentralization occur in both nations, with important roles played by regional governments and the voluntary sector leading to geographic diversity in the provision of health services. As is discussed below, the patterns for social services for the aged are even more diffuse.

Social Services for the Aged

Table 2, "Federalism and Social Services for the Aged in Canada and the United States," provides an overview of home- and community-based nonmedical services that help the aged remain functional in a variety of settings. The social service needs of the aged have been identified as a national issue in both countries and in-

Table 2.
FEDERALISM AND SOCIAL SERVICES FOR THE AGED IN CANADA AND THE UNITED STATES

	CANADA	UNITED STATES
NATIONAL	Greater emphasis on in home care Joint funding with provinces for the needy (CAP) Capped block grants to provinces: general assistance, emergency services for aged and disabled in community Joint committee with provinces on long term care services Specific responsibility for veterans (low income), Indians, territories	More emphasis on in home, community based care Tax exemptions for non-profit organizations Block grants (means tested) to states for social services (not age specific) Older Americans Act funds to states (population based; aged 60+) National demonstration programs Specific responsibility for veterans (low income), native Americans, territories
REGIONAL (PROVINCE/ STATE)	Joint funding with national government for the needy (CAP) Administer programs, determine level of cost sharing Some have demonstration projects to foster volunteer, community efforts Some regulate for-profit service delivery Some home care, case management insured	Broad discretion about services offered, recipient groups Some experiments in support for non-profits, family caregivers Can add own source funding, create new types of programs (e.g. day care) Provide funds to voluntary, non-profits to deliver social services Consumer protection regulation

LOCAL	Some administer CAP programs Some fund part of home support services Some receive provincial grants for meal services, day care	Receive federal funding via state agencies, state funding Delivery of social welfare programs, special services (e.g. guardianship) Regulation of facilities
FOR-PROFIT	Growing market, but still minor	Growing market, especially private care managers Some corporate sponsorship of community based services
NON-PROFIT	Old age groups can receive grants for community programs Support for family caregivers (respite)	Provision of services often on a contractual basis, own funding Support of community-based services (e.g. foundations, United Way) Support for family caregivers (respite)
FAMILIES, FRIENDS	Provide 85-90% of domiciliary care Can receive provincial payment on "exception" basis, some respite	Provide 80% of care, some respite Receive limited tax deductions for caregiving, direct pay experiments

home care is emphasized, largely because of the costs of institutional care. Responsibilities for social services are allocated among the three levels of government and the nongovernmental sector.

Federal revenues are allocated to promote regional government activity in providing social services to *needy persons, regardless of age,* via block grants to the regional governments–the Canadian Assistance Plan (CAP) and the Social Services Block Grant (SSBG) in the United States. These grants set broad guidelines permitting high levels of discretion as to which services are to be offered, and to whom. In addition, regional governments may finance a wide range of services with their own resources. Under CAP, the central government pays 50% of the cost to provinces of providing social assistance to persons in need and 50% of certain costs of providing welfare services, especially residential programs, to those likely to become in need. CAP tends to benefit most of those provinces that can best afford to implement programs and can also establish cost-sharing agreements with municipalities (Kane & Kane, 1985, 1989). Under the SSBG program, states receive funds on the basis of their population, within a federal expenditure ceiling, for services such as homemaker, chore, and personal care (U.S. Senate, 1988). States can engage local governments in these service delivery programs; many serve a high proportion of the aged relative to other age groups (Brown, 1990).

In the United States, however, a nonmeans-tested program is specifically targeted to persons aged 60 and over. Funds are provided to State Units on Aging–many of which were created via federal incentives–for allocation based on a statewide plan to Area Agencies on Aging, which were established in a similar fashion. As noted earlier, national-level agencies devoted to the aged have been created in both nations, with a customary focus on social services and largely responsible for ensuring the delivery of social services to indigenous populations, sometimes by providing subsidies or grants to representative nonprofit associations.

In both nations, the responsibility of regional governments in the realm of social services is somewhat more removed than in the health area; regional governments are far less likely to be involved in direct service delivery and administration, and prefer to provide funding and other incentives to local governments or voluntary organizations to discharge those tasks. The nature of financing mechanisms leads to geographic differences in the types of services provided (Brown, 1990; Health and Welfare Canada, 1990), as does the participation or lack of it by local governments, philanthropic organizations, and consumer groups. Local governments also receive direct or indirect funding from the two central governments for particular services; large cities may add their own programs, thereby increasing geographic differences in the availability of and access to services. Thus, regional and local governments and private agencies are seen as sharing the responsibility for financing and providing home-based services.

The United States has a more developed commercial provision of social services for the aged, especially for-profit case management for frail, and usually affluent, elders. There is also a strong tradition of corporate and foundation charitable activities, undergirded by preferential tax treatment. In both nations, however, the voluntary sector is heavily relied upon to provide social services, using public-sector funding and resources raised by their own efforts, resulting in even greater variability.

In summary, national and regional governments in the two nations try to promote the development of social services for needy persons, including the aged, through public funding to other governments and the nonprofit sector, with greater activity usually occurring at the regional level. In the United States, however, age-specific programs have also been created, and the commercial sector is gradually expanding its role. The voluntary nonprofit sector is especially important in both countries, in delivering and financing a wide range of services. Even more important is the role of families and friends in providing assistance, care, and support to enhance the well-being of frail elders; roughly 80% of all care is provided by this crucial group of informal caregivers in both nations.

Caregivers and Public Policy

Caregivers of the aged include spouses, adult children, siblings, grandchildren, and/or friends and neighbors (NACA, 1990b; Stone & Kemper, 1989). The nontemporary tasks they undertake are characterized by different levels of involvement: hands-on (e.g., household and some medical services, social assistance), paid care financed by the caregiver, and a combination of paid and informal care, often in co-residency arrangements (Chappell, 1990; Doty, 1986). In both nations, the family has primary responsibility for dependent care, which is seen as normative, as the right thing to do (Barusch, 1991; Hooyman, 1990; NACA, 1990b).

Unpaid family care is also seen as less costly and therefore more efficient. It is viewed as being of higher quality than formal care because of the emotional reciprocity, greater flexibility of hours, and lesser likelihood of caregiver turnover. It also provides access to care in underserved areas (Rivlin & Wiener, 1988). These views have resulted in the welfare of family caregivers not being a major goal of public policy. Public policymakers are reluctant to increase resources to support the family unless net savings are achieved in public expenditures (Barusch, 1991; Biegel, Schulz, Shore, & Morycz, 1989; Doty, 1986; Health and Welfare Canada, 1990; Hooyman, 1990). Until fairly recently, the rights of caregivers to public support have been minimally acknowledged in health and social service policies, and little has been done to prepare families for their long-term care obligations or to direct services to them (Barusch, 1991; Chappell, 1990; Hooyman, 1990, Kaye & Applegate, 1990; NACA, 1990a, 1990b; Stone, 1991). While complementarity of the institutional, community-based, and informal care systems is valued, government is unwilling to step in unless family resources or providers are absent (Biegel et al., 1989; Borgatta & Montgomery, 1987; Health and Welfare Canada, 1990; NACA, 1990a; Qureshi & Walker, 1986).

In both nations, central government programs do little to help caregivers *directly*. The bulk of programs in income security, health and social services, and housing are targeted to the older individual; families are assisted *indirectly* through reduction of the financial and caregiving burdens, often through the mechanism of social insurance. Canadian and American policymakers at both the national and regional levels, however, are concerned that too much assistance to the aged will result in the overuse of paid formal services and the abdication by families of their caregiving responsibility (Biegel et al., 1989; Chappell, 1990; Health and Welfare Canada, 1990; Kaye & Applegate, 1990; Linsk et al., 1992). Thus, policymakers in both nations are faced with complex policy objectives—they are attempting to develop services for older persons while at the same time they are encouraging family members to increase or maintain levels of caregiving, and seeking to ensure that families will not opt for more formal care use or "drop out" entirely. In addition, policymakers must decide if assistance should be provided universally or on a restricted basis.

Because of characteristic devolution to the provinces and increased decentralization to the states, policymakers at the regional level in both nations have been more active and often more innovative in constructing policies designed to meet some of the objectives delineated above. Table 3, "Provincial and State Programs to Assist Family Caregivers," provides an overview of the kinds of programs provided by North American regional governments that are supportive of family caregiving; service options such as home health and respite care, and caregiver training and counseling; and financial incentives such as direct payment and vouchers (Doty, 1986; Pillemer, MacAdam, & Wolf, 1989; Rivlin & Wiener, 1988).

Comparisons between Canada and the United States are hampered by the lack of data or incomplete information (e.g., on the status of family-leave legislation in Canada and state-level promotion of corporate eldercare programs in the United States); similarly, some programs in one nation simply do not exist in the other (e.g., private long-term care insurance exists in the United States, but not in Canada.). There is wide variation in programs both within and between the two countries; only home health care is uniformly offered, thereby supplementing the efforts of family caregivers; but in the United States, these services are limited under Medicare and are means-tested under Medicaid. Personal care programs that relieve caregivers of some of their responsibilities are fairly widespread for low-income recipients. Additionally, many regional governments in both nations have created task forces or commissions to study long-term care issues, with some attention paid to caregiver needs; in the United States, many have focused more specifically on Alzheimer's disease. In Canada, an intergovernmental commission on long-term care has complemented the work of single provincial government studies.

Other programs in the two nations that are fairly widespread and serve both caregivers and care recipients are day care and day

Table 3.
PROVINCIAL AND STATE PROGRAMS TO ASSIST FAMILY CAREGIVERS

PROGRAM	CANADA	UNITED STATES
Assess caregiver needs	1	ND
Caregiver training, counseling	3	30[a]
Case management	ND	32[b]
Day care/day health	4	36
Day hospital	2	ND
Direct payment to family members	2[c]	37
Family leave	ND	20
Home care/home health	10	50[b]
Home supportive services for caregiver	6	ND
Hospice	ND	9
Individual Medical Accounts (IMAs)	0	2
Long-term care insurance purchase promotion	0	4
Personal care	6	40
Promote corporate eldercare	ND	5
Respite care	7[d]	23[b]
Study commissions	4[e]	18[f] 24[a]
Tax credits	0	16
Vouchers	0	4

[a] Primarily related to Alzheimer's disease   [c] Others on "exception" basis   [e] Includes 1 Intergovernmental   ND No Data
[b] Usually via Medicaid waivers   [d] Requires minimal co-payment   [f] Long-term care specifically

Sources: American Association of Retired Persons, 1989; Biegel et al., 1989; Health and Welfare Canada, 1990; Kane & Kane, 1985; Lammers & Liebig, 1990; Linsk et al., 1992.

health care; day hospitals, however, are available only in Canada, but solely in two provinces. These programs can be especially beneficial for employed caregivers, a group about which there is increasingly greater concern (Biegel et al., 1989; NACA, 1990b). Corporate eldercare programs for employees appear to be even less widespread in Canada than they are in the United States, and governmental promotion of these efforts has not been substantial (Liebig, 1990; NACA, 1990b). Twenty states have enacted family-leave laws to help employees with their caregiving responsibilities, but the majority of these have not focused on eldercare concerns.

Fewer programs exist that directly assist caregivers in either nation. Government-sponsored respite care to give caregivers some relief is fairly widespread in 70% of the provinces and 46% of the states. Caregiver training and counseling, which help caregivers develop coping and care skills, are supported by a large number of states, but with a major emphasis on the needs of Alzheimer's caregivers; few provinces are so engaged. On the other hand, a majority of the provinces have targeted some home support services specifically to caregivers, and one assesses the specific needs of caregivers (Health and Welfare Canada, 1990).

Financial assistance is an approach more frequently used in the United States than in Canada, where a number of needed services are provided on a more universal basis in several provinces (Kane & Kane, 1985; Health and Welfare Canada, 1990). Nearly a third of the states offer tax credits to help employed family caregivers, similar to the national Dependent Care Assistance Program (DCAP), but co-residency is often required and higher-income families are the major beneficiaries (Biegel et al., 1989; Rivlin & Wiener, 1988). A handful of states have used vouchers for certain services and for partial assistance for long-term care insurance purchase.

Direct payment to family caregivers by regional governments to relieve some financial burdens has been more widespread in the United States. In Canada, only two provinces have such a program for low-income families; others allow this only if no other caregivers are available (Health and Welfare Canada, 1990). By contrast, 37 states provide some direct payment to family members, but under highly restricted conditions, with the main constraint being Medicaid kinship rules (Linsk et al., 1992). There is wide variation in the states' interpretations of those rules, however, as was evidenced in the early 1980s by only a few states trying to enforce Health Care Finance Administration (HCFA) guidelines on family responsibility (Lammers & Klingman, 1984a), and by only 15 states now disallowing payments to spouses (Linsk et al., 1992). Other restrictions, some based on state statutes and regulations, include co-residency and the requirement that caregivers relinquish outside employment if they are compensated for caregiving. As documented by Nathan Linsk and colleagues (1992), these restrictions have increased within the last five years.

It is clear that both Canadian and American caregivers receive limited direct assistance, which is largely dependent on their geographic location, and that regional government sovereignty drives long-term care policy. In the United States, however, HCFA restricts state discretion (Linsk et al., 1992). By contrast, the provinces have had greater leeway to develop more services specifically tailored to caregivers, reflecting the more universal approach of the Canadian system; the states are more focused on the development of nonpublic ways of financing care, in keeping with the U.S. emphasis on cost containment and cost shifting. In addition, the states direct many of their efforts to Alzheimer's caregivers, rather than more broadly. Direct payment policies in both nations, while somewhat more widespread than a decade ago, are still highly restricted, reflecting a lack of consensus about what constitutes an appropriate "sharing" of the caregiving function between families and government. In addition, the increased tying of caregiver assistance to health policy, which perhaps garners more financial involvement from the national government, runs the risk of "medicalizing" this help and heightening the tensions between the national and regional governments, as they grapple with the issues of long-term care–separately and jointly–for a larger, much older population (Lammers & Liebig, 1990; NACA, 1991).

The Future of Federalism
and Care for the Aged

Federalism is in a state of flux in both countries. In Canada, political debates over the past decade have revolved around the need to redesign the Canadian constitution and strengthen further the roles of the provinces and indigenous populations, so as to keep Canada united (Burgess, 1990; Russell, 1990). Proposals have included changing the upper house in the national legislature to represent the provinces, similar to the U.S. system. While a rewriting of the U.S. Constitution has not been proposed as a resolution to intergovernmental tensions, Alice Rivlin (1992) among others has called for a clearer distinction between the responsibilities of national and state governments, with the federal government broadening social insurance to include basic health insurance, the states being responsible for a "productivity agenda," and a new system of common, shared taxes to put state financing on a more secure and equal footing, similar to the Canadian system.

These continuing shifts in federalism in both nations will affect family caregivers and the persons for whom they are caring. Even if the projected reductions in the numbers of caregivers are accurate, families will remain a critical, if not *the* crucial, component in long-term care. How either society will respond to caregiver needs depends, in part, on the willingness of those informal care providers to be advocates for long-term care reform (Stone & Kemper, 1989). If family caregiving policy is to evolve, this advocacy must be carried out at both the national and regional government levels, and especially at the latter level where policies affecting family caregivers will continue to dominate.

In each country, we currently have a family caregiving policy by default, much of it unsupportive of family efforts. Given the concerns about government supplanting the family and philosophies about the "rightness" of family care, an emphasis should be placed on those policies that empower families. These can include assessing caregiver needs and training caregivers to carry out their tasks more capably, by consulting with them about needed services (NACA, 1990b) rather than only relying on the judgment of professional caregivers and by providing them with "one-stop" up-to-date information and referral to existing services. Consideration should be given to paying family members, at least on an "exception" basis, when other appropriate caregivers do not exist (e.g., for situations where care needs to be culturally sensitive care or is not available in rural areas). In addition, based on the premise that family caregiving is both a private and social good (Biegel et al., 1989; Linsk et al., 1992), task forces at the regional level should examine current public policies (national and regional) that act as barriers to family care (such as housing codes) and that provide a basic level of assistance and services to all family caregivers (for instance, Saskatchewan's home care districts program). Task forces should also examine important equity issues, for example, whether it is fair to require relatives to provide services that governments would give to those without family (Doty, 1986; Linsk et al., 1992; Rivlin & Wiener, 1988; Wiener & Hanley, 1992), and other value concerns.

Finally, both countries need studies of what interventions best support families. Research thus far is relatively inconclusive as to what kinds of supportive policies are most effective for different kinds of caregivers (Barusch, 1991; Biegel et al., 1989; Doty, 1986; Linsk et al., 1992; Pillemer, MacAdam & Wolf, 1989; Qureshi & Walker, 1986). Without this information to guide policymakers at both regional and national levels, a more rational and appropriate redefinition of who should care for the aged will not be articulated.

REFERENCES

American Association of Retired Persons. (1989). *State policy status report no. 4: Long-term care programs and policies*. Washington, DC: AARP.

Barusch, A.S. (1991). *Elder care: Family training and support*. Newbury Park, CA: Sage.

Bickerton, J. (1990). Atlantic Canada: The dynamics of dependence in a federal system. In M. Burgess (Ed.), *Canadian federalism: Past, present and future* (pp. 120-144). New York: Leicester University.

Biegel, D.E., Schulz, R. Shore, B.K., & Morycz, R. (1989). Economic support for family caregivers of the elderly: Public sector policies. In M.Z. Goldstein (Ed.), *Family involvement in treatment of the elderly* (pp. 159-201). New York: American Psychiatric Press.

Bloksberg, L.M. (1989). Intergovernmental relations: Change and continuity. *Journal of Aging & Social Policy, 1* (3/4), 11-36.

Borgatta, E.F., & Montgomery, R.J.V. (1987). Aging, policy and societal values. In E.F. Borgatta and R.J.V. Montgomery (Eds.), *Critical issues in aging policy: Linking research and values* (pp. 7-27). Newbury Park, CA: Sage.

Bowman, A. O'M., & Pagano, M.A. (1990). The state of American federalism, 1989-1990. *Publius, 20* (3), 1-26.

Brink, S. (1992). Supportive housing for the frail elderly in Canada. Paper presented at a conference on Housing Policies for Frail Older Persons: International Perspectives and Prospects, Los Angeles, February 20-22.

Brown, H.W. (1990). *A survey of the states on the Title XX social services block grant program.* Washington, DC: AARP.

Burgess, M. (1990). Canadian imperialism as nationalism: The legacy and significance of the imperial federation movement in Canada. In M. Burgess (Ed.), *Canadian federalism: Past, present and future* (pp. 60-78). New York: Leicester University.

Chandler, W., & Bakvis, H. (1989). Federalism and the strong-state/weak-state conundrum: Canadian economic policymaking in comparative perspective. *Publius, 19* (1), 59-70.

Chappell, N. (1990). Aging and social care. In R. Binstock and L.K. George (Eds.), *Handbook of aging and the social sciences* (3rd edition) (pp. 438-454). New York: Academic Press.

Doty, P. (1986). Family care of the elderly: The role of public policy. *Milbank Quarterly, 64* (1), 34-75.

Dye, T. (1990). *American federalism: Competition among governments.* Lexington, MA: D.C. Heath.

Hanson, R.L. (1990). Intergovernmental relations. In V. Gray, H. Jacob and R. Albritton (Eds.), *Politics in the American states: A comparative analysis* (5th ed) (pp. 38-81). Glenview, IL: Scott Foresman.

Health and Welfare Canada, Federal/Provincial/Territorial Committee on Long-Term Care (1990). *Description of long-term care services in provinces and territories of Canada.* Ottawa: Health and Welfare Canada.

Hooyman, N.R. (1990). Women as caregivers of the elderly: Implications for social welfare policy and practice. In D.E. Biegel and A. Blum (Eds.), *Aging and caregiving: Theory, research and policy* (pp. 221-241). Newbury Park, CA: Sage.

Kane, R.A., & Kane, R.L. (1989). Long-term care for the elderly in Canada. In T. Schwab (Ed.), *Caring for an aging world: International models for long-term care, financing and delivery* (pp. 193-210). New York: McGraw-Hill Information Services.

Kane, R.L., & Kane, R.A. (1985). *A will and a way: What the United States can learn from Canada about caring for the elderly.* New York: Columbia University.

Kaye, L.W., & Applegate, J.S. (1990). *Men as caregivers to the elderly: Understanding and aiding unrecognized family support.* Lexington, MA: D.C. Heath.

Lammers, W.W., & Klingman, D. (1984a). Family responsibility laws and state politics: Adoption patterns and policy implications (mimeo).

Lammers, W.W., & Klingman, D. (1984b). *State policies and the aging: source, trends, and options.* Lexington, MA: D.C. Heath.

Lammers, W.W., & Liebig, P.S. (1990). State health policies, federalism and the elderly. *Publius, 20* (3), 131-148.

Landes, R.G. (1983). *The Canadian polity.* Scarborough, ONT: Prentice Hall Canada.

Leach, R.H. (1981). *Studies in comparative federalism: Australia, Canada, the United States and West Germany.* Washington, D.C.: U.S. Advisory Commission on Intergovernmental Relations.

Liebig, P.S. (1990). Employer initiatives in long-term care. In P.S. Liebig and W.W. Lammers (Eds.), *California policy choices for long-term care* (pp. 75-97). Los Angeles: Andrus Gerontology Center.

Linsk, N.L., Keigher, S.M., Simon-Rusinowitz, L., & England, S.E. (1992). *Wages for caring: Compensating family care of the elderly.* New York: Praeger.

Lipset, S.M. (1991). Canada and the United States: The great divide. *Current History, 90* (560), 432-7.

Marmor, T.R. (1991). Canada's health care system: A model for the United States? *Current History, 90* (560), 422-7.

Moroney, R.M. (1986). *Shared responsibility: Families and social policy.* New York: Aldene Press.

Nathan, R.P. (1990). Federalism–The great "composition." In A. King (Ed.), *The new American political system* (2nd version) (pp. 231-261). Washington, DC: American Enterprise Institute.

National Advisory Council on Aging (1990a). *Community services in health care for seniors.* Ottawa: Minister of Supply and Services Canada.

National Advisory Council on Aging (1990b). *The NACA position on informal caregiving: Support and enhancement.* Ottawa: Minister of Supply and Services Canada.

National Advisory Council on Aging (1991). *Intergovernmental relations and the aging of the population: Challenges facing Canada.* Ottawa: Minister of Supply and Services Canada.

Pillemer, K., MacAdam, M.Y., & Wolf, R.S. (1989). Services to families with dependent elders. *Journal of Aging & Social Policy, 1* (3/4), 67-88.

Presthus, R. (1974). *Elites in the policy process.* New York: Cambridge University Press.

Qureshi, H., & Walker, A. (1986). Caring for elderly people. In C. Phillipson and A. Walker (Eds.), *Aging and social policy: A critical assessment* (pp. 109-127). Brookfield, VT: Gower.

Rivlin, A. (1992). A new vision of American federalism. *Public Administration Review, 52,* 315-320.

Rivlin, A., & Wiener, J.M. (1988). *Caring for the disabled elderly: Who will pay?* Washington, DC: Brookings Institution.

Russell, P.A. (1990). The jurisdictional pendulum within Canadian federalism. In M. Burgess (Ed.), *Canadian federalism: Past, present and future* (pp. 40-59). New York: Leicester University.

Stevenson, G. (1985). The division of powers. In R. Simeon (Ed.), *Division of powers and public policy* (pp. 71-123). Toronto: University of Toronto.

Stone, R. (1991). Familial obligations: Issues for the 1990s. *Generations, 15* (3), 47-50.

Stone, R.I. & Kemper, P. (1989). Spouses and children of disabled elders: How large a constituency for long-term care reform? *Milbank Quarterly, 67* (3/4), 485-506.

U.S. Senate, Special Committee on Aging (1988). *Home care at the crossroads.* Washington, D.C.: U.S. Government Printing Office.

Van Horn, C. (1989). The quiet revolution. In C. Van Horn (Ed.), *The state of the states* (pp. 3-15). Washington, D.C.: Congressional Quarterly Press.

Wagenberg, R., Soderlund, W., Nelson, R., & Briggs, D. (1990). Federal societies and the founding of federal states: An examination of the origins of Canadian confederation. In M. Burgess (Ed.), *Canadian federalism: Past, present and future* (pp. 7-39). New York: Leicester University.

Watts, R.L. (1990). The Macdonald Commission and Canadian federalism. In M. Burgess (Ed.), *Canadian federalism: Past, present and future* (pp. 155-175). New York: Leicester University.

Wiener, J.M., & Hanley, R.J. (1992). Caring for the disabled elderly: There's no place like home. In S.M. Shortell & U.E. Reinhardt (Eds.), *Improving health policy and management: Nine critical research issues for the 1990s* (pp. 75-110). Ann Arbor, MI: Health Administration Press.

Zimmerman, J.F. (1991). *Federal preemption: The silent revolution.* Ames, IA: Iowa State University Press.

Implications of Shifting
Health Care Policy
for Caregiving in Canada

Neena L. Chappell, PhD

University of Victoria
British Columbia, Canada

SUMMARY. The health care system in Canada, like other industrialized countries, is undergoing a questioning and a change unlike any it has seen for many decades. This article begins with a brief description of the Canadian health care system, then discusses the shifts taking place in health care policy, the assumptions behind these shifts, and the choices that are being made. The current debate draws on knowledge about seniors and their caregivers. The shifts also have implications for caregiving, and these are examined. It is concluded that the new vision of an appropriate health care system that is emerging provides opportunity for greater recognition of and participation by caregivers. At the same time, however, it holds the danger that the burden of care will be shifted even more to their shoulders. It is not yet clear which direction it is going to take.

Virtually all industrialized nations, certainly in Western Europe and North America, are in crisis over health care costs. As noted by

---

Neena L. Chappell is the first Director of the Centre on Aging at the University of Victoria. She was Founding Director of the Research Centre on Aging at the University of Manitoba. Dr. Chappell has published extensively in the areas of health, health care, informal caregiving, and social policy for seniors.

[Haworth co-indexing entry note]: "Implications of Shifting Health Care Policy for Caregiving in Canada," Chappell, Neena L. Co-published simultaneously in the *Journal of Aging & Social Policy,* (The Haworth Press, Inc.) Vol. 5, No. 1/2, 1993, pp. 39-55; and: *International Perspectives on State and Family Support for the Elderly* (ed: Scott A. Bass and Robert Morris) The Haworth Press, Inc., 1993, pp. 39-55. Multiple copies of this article/chapter may be purchased from The Haworth Document Delivery Center [1-800-3-HAWORTH; 9:00 a.m. - 5:00 p.m. (EST)].

39

Robert Evans and Gregg Stoddart (1990), the perception of a cost crisis exists irrespective of the type of health care delivery system found in the country or the amount spent on health care. This conflict is developing as paying agencies attempt to limit the increase in resources provided to the health care system. The crisis has not escaped Canada. The percent of GNP spent on health care in Canada (9% in 1987) is higher than the average 7.3% for Organization for Economic Cooperation and Development-member countries in the same year. On a per capita basis, Canada has the second most expensive system in the world, second only to the United States. Stated differently, Canada spends more on health per capita than any industrialized country that has national health insurance.

A questioning of the health care system has been coincident with the cost crisis. The reasons for it are similar in Canada to those expressed in other industrialized nations. Cumulative international evidence exists as to the ineffective, inefficient, and unevaluated portions of health care activity (McPherson, 1990). With this is rising concern that medicine cannot do more, or can do little more, to increase health, that is, there are many modern-day ills that medicine cannot cure. This is particularly evident among an aging population where chronic disabilities rather than acute infectious diseases prevail. There is also increased acceptance of a broader health promotion perspective within the population generally. The coalescing of these factors has resulted in a questioning of both the efficiency and effectiveness of existing health care systems throughout developed nations.

Discussions taking place about the health care system and resultant policy changes not only draw on knowledge about seniors and caregivers to seniors but also have implications for both groups. This article begins with a brief description of the Canadian health care system. It then discusses the shifts taking place in health care policy, assumptions behind these shifts, and the choices that are being made. The implications of this shifting health care policy for caregiving in Canada are then examined. This is a time of change, and future directions within the health care system are not yet clear.

CANADA'S HEALTH CARE SYSTEM

Canada's health care system, like those in many European countries, provides universal access to physician services and acute hospital care. Health is a provincial responsibility, but the federal government was instrumental in establishing the universal medical care program through its command of monetary resources and its ability to set national standards and priorities. Initially, the federal government matched every dollar the provinces spent on approved services, but in the late 1970s this was changed to a system of cash grants (block funding). There is a single funding source (government, and ultimately the taxpayer) but Canada does not have socialized medical care. Most health care resources are in the private sector. Physicians work on a fee-for-service basis for themselves, not for the government. Fees are negotiated between provincial governments and medical associations. Hospitals are private nonprofit organizations. In 1984 the Canada Health Act prevented user charges or extra billing from being levied.

Community-based programs are not covered by any comprehensive national insurance scheme. They have tended to develop as add-ons to existing institutional medical care. The lack of a national insurance scheme for home care services is demonstrated by the lack of uniformity from province to province. Indeed, only recently has there been a national compilation that describes the long-term care services available throughout the country (Health and Welfare Canada, 1991). Some provinces provide certain services (such as chiropody) as part of their home care program, others do not. In one province, certain services are offered at no fee to the client, but there may be a charge in another. Some provinces still require physician referral for home care, others do not. Manitoba exemplifies one of the more progressive provinces, with a universal home care program that is a part of their universal health care system. Referral can be from anyone, and there is an independent assessment by a nurse or a social worker. Long-term institutional care (nursing home care), like home care, may or may not be covered under a provincial program, varying from jurisdiction to jurisdiction.

Medicare locked in established patterns of service delivery. Until recently there have been few efforts to either find more cost-effective means of delivering services or assess effectiveness in terms of health outcomes. Of late there has been increasing concern over the continually escalating cost of health care, which appears to have no limit, and the lack of adequate knowledge about the effectiveness of this care in terms of health outcomes. Indeed, the focus of most provincial policies to date has been expenditure control (Muldoon & Stoddart, 1989). The general solution for controlling costs has been to stop building hospitals and hospital additions, and to decrease the acquisition of new technology. There has been some effort to restrict enrollment in medical schools to limit the supply of physicians. At the time of writing, a newly announced report to the federal and all provincial Ministries of Health has recommended decreasing entrance to medical schools further (Barer & Stoddart, 1991).

Provinces have also resorted to reduced increases, no increases, or in some instances small decreases to hospital budgets. Hospitals in Canada are private nonprofit organizations, as mentioned, that operate with global budgets (excluding funds for medical technologies). There have also been efforts to put global caps on physicians' salaries negotiated at the aggregate level. One also sees some effort to reduce the numbers of procedures that are eligible for payment within the national insurance scheme.

The federal government's concern was evident in the 1970s resulting in the change in funding from a matching dollar basis to block funding. However, in 1986 that legislation was amended to reduce the rate of growth of federal contributions further. Additional reductions were announced in 1989 and 1990. Beginning in 1995-1996, growth will be restricted still further (National Council on Welfare, 1990). The newly passed Bill C-69 will see federal transfer payments to the provinces reduced to nil, and the provinces' taxing powers increased in order to make up for this loss. Such a course removes any power the federal government had in the Canada Health Act of 1984 to prevent provinces from charging user fees or extra billing (that Act permits the federal government to reduce its transfer payments to the provinces by an amount equal to that raised by such means). Bill C-69 removes much of the national ability to ensure comparable services from province to province, and it also smooths the way for the economically disadvantaged provinces to offer inferior health care services.

Recent Developments

Recently, during the 1990s, there has been evident change in the attitude towards the health care system by provincial ministries of health. There is now much greater effort to reduce costs and to drastically change the health care system. Virtually every province has established inquiries, commissions, or other committees to examine cost inefficiencies within their health care systems. In Ontario there is the Premier's Commission on Health; in British Columbia there has been a Royal Commission on Health; Manitoba has just released a Reform Document on Health Care. Collectively, the Ministers of Health, including the federal Minister, have commissioned a report to examine the health care system. One of the reasons for this shift has been increasing cumulative evidence questioning the role of medicine as a precise science within the health care system.

Evidence of unexplained variations in medical practice and in appropriate clinical policies constitute part of this research (Lomas, 1990). Unexplained variation in surgical rates, for example, point to the discretionary nature of medicine. In the province of Manitoba, Evelyn Shapiro (1991) reports variations in surgical rates between areas of the province, differences of opinion among physicians selecting patients for elective surgery, underestimation of risk and possible overestimation of benefits associated with some procedures, the adoption of new procedures before the risks and benefits are thoroughly studied, and physician practice style as well as the way physicians deal with medical uncertainty as major contributors to the differences in hospital admission rates between geographic areas. International research has demonstrated that between 15% and 30% of medical services are inappropriate (Lomas, 1990 cited in Barer & Stoddart, 1991). While there may be disagreement on the precise rates, there is no longer any question that some portion of medical intervention is unnecessary, inefficient, or produces small returns.

At the same time, there is increasing recognition that medicine may be reaching its limits and spending more on health care will not necessarily enhance the health of people in various nations but will leave fewer dollars for other health-enhancing activities. Increasingly, documentation of the role of nonmedical factors in health is being accepted. For example, the role of income and social class (the economically disadvantaged are also more disadvantaged in terms of their health) now enjoys widespread acceptance. The greatest predictor of ill health is poverty. Similarly, the importance of social support for maintaining health is also largely undisputed. As James Lubben and associates (1989) have noted, the relationship between social networks and hospitalization is as strong as the relationship between smoking and mortality that led to the Surgeon General's warning on cigarette packages many years ago.

A recent United States study (General Accounting Office, 1991) notes that only 10% of premature deaths are attributable to inadequate health services. The rest are due to unhealthy lifestyles (50%), environmental factors (20%), and human biological factors (20%). Studies demonstrating the importance of the overall host response (i.e., individual total response unexplained by any particular system, such as the immune system) are also available. For example, a 15-year study shows the strongest predictor of longevity is work satisfaction and overall happiness, exceeding the contribution of other factors such as diet, exercise, medical care, or genetic inheritance (cited in Berliner, 1977). The documentation and acceptance of nonmedical factors as contributors to our health has led to a questioning of the role of additional expenditures in our current health care system where physicians exercise the majority of control. The growing acceptance of nonmedical factors in health is evident at both the political and populous levels in the increasing popularity of health promotion or lifestyle approaches to maintaining health.

The policy shifts taking place in health care reflect a strong concern on the part of governments, in particular ministries of health, about stabilizing if not decreasing their health care budgets. The growing documentation and acceptance of a critical appraisal of the role of physicians and the medical bias within the system provide fertile ground for a vision of a less expensive health care system. The extent to which the current political willingness to change policy is driven primarily by cost concerns while utilizing cumulative research and knowledge to save dollars or the extent to which there is genuine interest in enhancing a healthy population through less medical, more community approaches to health is not known.

Irrespective of the motivation, the forces are coalescing to lead to the most profound changes the health care system has seen in Canada since the implementation of universal hospital insurance in 1957, followed by universal physician insurance in 1968. It is now well recognized that we have health *care* policy, rather than health policy; that medicine has a bias towards intervention that is not always warranted; that Canadian hospitals have few incentives for tracking cost per patient day or cost per case; and that physicians bear no cost for utilizing and therefore "creating" the cost for hospitals. In summary, those who pay for the health care system want it to be both more cost-effective and more efficient. Cumulative evidence in favor of community-based care suggests these two goals could be compatible in a drastically altered health care system. Seniors and caregivers play an important role in helping to shape this new vision.

SENIORS AND THEIR CAREGIVERS

Part of the argument for the redistribution of health care dollars is that seniors and others prefer to stay in their own homes (Habitat, 1989; Province of British Columbia, 1991); they choose home care over institutional care. The two most preferred options among British Columbian seniors are home care in their own homes or apartment living with services available (Baker, 1987).

Furthermore, some of the failures of the existing Medicare system are most evident when examining its appropriateness in relation to old age. This is because the major illnesses of old age are chronic conditions or acute flareups of chronic conditions rather than acute diseases. The most common chronic illnesses among seniors in Canada are arthritis or rheumatism (55%), hypertension (39%), heart trouble (26%), and respiratory problems (24%) (Statistics Canada, 1988). The greatest need among seniors is for services that help them cope with chronic conditions and functional disabilities. Long-term care is often required.

The wealth of gerontological research on the support provided to seniors from the informal network also argues in favor of long-term community care (Antonucci, 1990; Chappell, 1992). The predominance of informal caregiving over use of the formal care system is now well established. Robert L. Kane and associates (1990) note that irrespective of whether a country provides comprehensive health insurance, between 75% and 85% of all personal care received by seniors comes from the informal network. Family and friends are the first resort for care to elders; they provide the vast majority of that care; and it is the lack of informal support, not ill health, that is the main predictor of long-term institutionalization. Despite any changes taking place in society such as increased divorce rates and more women working in paid labor, the informal network remains the mainstay of care for seniors. Furthermore, establishment of formal home care programs does not discourage informal care provision but can prolong it (Horowitz, Sherman, & Durmanskin, 1983; Noelker & Poulshock, 1982). Families by and large want to provide care.

The care received from the informal network has not gone unnoticed. These arguments help provide an alternative vision of a less costly health care system. It is too early to tell the extent to which or the form in which the vision will be implemented. The implementation has the danger of falling far short of the promise. Current changes suggest reason for concern.

A typical response to escalating costs is to close long-term hospital beds without any expansion to home care programs. This is evident, for example, in Nova Scotia and in Newfoundland. Some provinces are taking a broader approach and arguing for the closure of institutional beds while simultaneously placing a greater emphasis on community social support. Ontario (with a total population of just over 9 million and an elderly population of 1,064,200 in 1988, Chambers, Labelle, Gafni, & Goeree, 1992) released a discussion paper arguing for just such a move. It is taking $67 million from the institutional sector and transferring it to community care over a one-year period. However, this constitutes only 1% of the institutional budget in that province.

Perhaps most impressive to date is the action plan for cost savings formulated by the government of Manitoba. Here many of the inefficiencies within the medical and institutional sectors are documented (Manitoba Health, 1992). There is an explicit and public recognition that our Medicare system has a bias towards the development of high-cost services and towards geographic centralization of services with expenditures focused in major urban areas. There is further both explicit and public recognition that global budgeting of hospitals allows the managing of expenditures but does not (at least as yet) provide systematic evaluations of the effectiveness of services or of care as measured by health outcome. This document calls for bed closures and for the explicit transference of medical and institutional dollars to an expansion of community care. In addition, it calls for the rigorous scientific evaluation of changes within the system as a monitoring device. It is too early to see whether the government will make all the changes of which it speaks.

In British Columbia, the now well-known Quick Response Team provides care in the home for individuals admitted to emergency wards of hospitals who do not require in-patient care. This concept is being implemented in other provinces. It has been evaluated and has been shown to cut down on hospital admissions. Accordingly, parts of the hospital budget have been transferred over to expand the Quick Response Team. However, increases in the budget have gone to the Quick Response Team per se and not to home care, which experiences increased demand as individuals move on to the home care program within a few days.

In other words, provinces share the strategy of the closure of beds and the narrowing of the medical sector in the particular directions in which they are moving. All provinces that have medical schools are looking at limiting enrollment, and there is experimentation with alternatives to fee-for-service payment schemes for physicians. However, provinces differ in the extent to which they are taking a total systems approach to reform, and the extent to which there is a recognized need to expand community home care services in order to provide needed care when institutional and medical services are cut back. Whether adequate home care services will be put in place is an open question.

Nevertheless, gerontology and gerontological research is particularly relevant for the changes that are occurring. The fact that seniors frequently require long-term care and prefer to receive it in the community together with the fact that this type of care is less costly has not escaped the attention of the provincial governments.

IMPLICATIONS FOR CAREGIVERS

The study of seniors and of caregivers is not only relevant in terms of the changes that are taking place and the new vision of health care that is emerging, the changes also have implications for both groups. Whether formal home care is adequately funded obviously has major implications for caregivers. If it is not, cutbacks in medical care will increase the demands on informal caregivers, a process that is happening in the United States (Estes & Wood, 1986). Reimbursement to hospitals based on DRG's (diagnostic-related groups) has lead to earlier discharge of patients, which results in greater demand on community care services. However, Medicare and Medicaid are becoming more medicalized so that fewer home care programs are eligible, placing more demands on informal caregivers. If medical care is cut back without an expansion of community care, seniors are left not with a new health care system, simply a less adequate old system. The danger of current arguments is that they will be used to diminish medical and institutional services without expanding home care services. These dangers are very real.

Even if home care is expanded, how this takes place has implications for caregivers. If current programs are simply expanded, caregivers have little say. They must adjust to the system if they want the older persons in their care to receive the services. Even though the informal care system is a much larger partner, it has been largely ignored by public policy, and has had to adapt silently to the advantages and constraints set by the public sector (Baldock & Evers, 1991). The new mixed economy of welfare now being recognized in Europe seeks to incorporate informal, voluntary, and private sectors with the public sector in the provision of care. This explicit recognition of the informal sector is new. All provinces in Canada recognize the need to provide services to caregivers (for example, respite care and support services); most recognize it explicitly at the policy level. The mixed economy of the welfare model goes beyond the provision of services to caregivers, recognizing them as partners in the care provision system. This new status can mean more power for the informal sector. It can also mean greater scrutiny by the public sector, that is, more state inspection. The shift from bureaucratic centralism to regulated pluralism means a greater role for caregivers. Sweden, the United Kingdom, and the Netherlands are pursuing explicit policies to integrate and coordinate public, commercial, voluntary, and informal forms of care. Canada is moving in the same direction but has not explicitly recognized this model. Nevertheless, the provincial governments are recognizing roles for informal caregivers, for the voluntary sector, and for the private sector that were not evident a few years ago.

Sweden, the United Kingdom, and the Netherlands are, however, simultaneously targeting those with highest need and lowest incomes for public care. This shifts the burden of care to informal caregivers, most of whom are women, because policies that are restrictive in a host of ways (for example, requiring medical certification, aimed at only those 80 and over, or aimed at the extremely frail) will leave substantial portions of seniors requiring care who must turn to family and friends or go without. Similarly, home care policies that provide care only as a substitute to informal care do not necessarily assist caregivers, depending on how they are implemented. If they are delivered to complement and prolong care provided by families, they can assist caregivers. If they are delivered only when families are not available, they may be of little assistance to caregivers.

The extent to which home care is viewed as part of the health care system or is viewed as a separate social care system also has implications for caregivers. Pamela Doty (1988) notes that in virtually all countries there is resistance to incorporating nonmedical long-term care services within the rubric of health programs. In most European countries, these services are characterized as social services and tend to be administered locally. In this respect Canada is different. Six of the 10 provinces (British Columbia, Alberta, Saskatchewan, Manitoba, Quebec, and Prince Edward Island) deliver home care services from their provincial departments of health. All other provinces and the Northwest Territories deliver at least some home care services through the department of health, with some through a department of community or social services and some delivered jointly by both departments (Health and Welfare Canada, 1991).

This willingness to accept home care, community services as part of the health care system is consistent with the debate in Canada that links reform of the universal Medicare system to enhanced community care services. In Canada, at least, it is not a question of a separate system. Rather, criticisms, questions, and assessments of the appropriateness of medical care and the dominance of physicians are part of the debate about reform within the system. This suggests the potential at least of reform, with a greater emphasis on community care and on nonmedical care. A recent federal committee (Porter, 1991) has recommended a shift from institutional services to community, home-care social-support services. It has further recommended the use of a wide range of health care professionals other than physicians within the insured health care system. Some provinces have taken a more active step in actually transferring dollars. As mentioned earlier, at the forefront of this move at the present time is Manitoba with its reform document.

Even if the home care system were expanded and caregivers were true participants in the decisionmaking process, we do not know what type of use they would make of services available to them. Research from the United States on utilization of such services points consistently to their low and judicious usage. Respite care is the service most frequently requested by informal caregivers (Heagerty, Dunn, & Watson, 1988), but utilization remains low (George, 1988). Only a small proportion of those deemed eligible actually use the service when it is offered. Linda George (1988) reports that fewer than 25% of caregivers use any type of formal services other than physician services. Younger adult caregivers, those with higher incomes, and those with more informal social support are more likely to use community services. Similarly, demand for support or self-help groups for caregivers is not high.

Several reasons have been suggested for this low rate of utilization. Caregivers wait until very late to utilize the services, indeed until the elder requires terminal care. It has also been argued that caregivers are unfamiliar with such services, and psychologically are conflicted over the appropriateness of asking for formal care to provide assistance with caring for a loved one (Saperstein, 1988). Others suggest that families under stress may have a limited picture of the future, and it is difficult for them to understand how services can assist them, or that caregivers may not perceive their own need, they may have negative attitudes towards receiving these services, they may fear loss of independence, and they may not understand bureaucratic structures (Rakowski & Clark, 1985; Scott & Roberto, 1985). In addition, structural barriers such as someone to care for the elder for them so that they can attend support groups and lack of transportation can also hinder usage (Gonyea, 1988).

CONCLUSIONS

Canada, like other industrialized nations, has spent the last decade recognizing and putting in place home care programs for elders. Toward the end of that period, Canadians were recognizing the role of others (family, friends, neighbors, and the community) in the well-being and provision of care for elders. The recognition of informal caregivers coincided with a perceived cost crisis within the health care system, and is now being used as part of the argument for reshaping universal Medicare. It offers the promise of a new vision, which appeals to governments as less expensive than high-tech medical care in hospitals. However, it requires a new role for caregivers, different from their role in the existing system in which they are treated separately from and largely ignored by the public sector.

The transition that is taking place calls for a change in some of the underlying assumptions to health care. Canada had accepted public responsibility for the nation's health, recognized when universal hospital insurance followed by universal physician insurance was put in place across the country. The passing of the Canada Health Act in 1984 to discourage user fees and extra billing was a further explicit acceptance that there should not be two systems of care based on one's ability to pay.

Canadians have proudly accepted this shared responsibility for the risks of health. This was evident in a recent survey comparing the satisfaction of Canadians, Americans, and the British with their health care systems (Blendon, 1989). Only 10%· of Americans believe their health care system works pretty well, while 27% of the British believe theirs does, and fully 56% (over half) of Canadians believe theirs does. On the other hand, fully 89% (the vast majority) of Americans believe that their health care system requires fundamental underlying change in terms of its direction and structure, 69% of the British believe this of their system, and less than half (42%) of Canadians believe this of their system.

Of the three countries studied, only Americans are so dissatisfied that they want to change their system for that of another country (29% would select the British system and 61% would select the Canadian system). Among the British, 28% would select the Canadian system and 12% the U.S. system. Only 5% of Canadians, by contrast, would select the British system and only 3% would choose the U.S. system–they overwhelmingly chose their own system.

The cost crisis, new knowledge, and changing values are leading to a questioning of the health care system, which includes a belief that medicine is not all there is to maintaining health. It has also lead to many questions about the willingness of Canadians to maintain a universal system that is very different from the one they have known. Even during this questioning there is no sense that the aged poor should go without. It is assumed that those who are disadvantaged economically will receive care and it shall be subsidized. In other words, the underlying principles of universal Medicare are not being questioned per se. However, the changes that are taking place have consequences for those underlying principles that are not always recognized. For example, if medicine is cut back and community care is not expanded, this will have obvious implications for health care. Those who cannot afford to pay will not have access to all of the services that others do.

The questioning and the changes taking place are threatening to vested interests, and battle lines are being drawn. Strikes by physicians and threats by their professional associations to charge for services that previously were not charged for (such as physical examinations and filling prescriptions over the phone) have been evident in more than one province. In those provinces (such as Ontario and Manitoba) whose governments have made their intention clear to start shifting health care resources away from the institutional sector to the community, the institutional sector is trying to extend its boundaries into the community. Hospitals and long-term care institutions are examining ways to tap into these community resources by providing outreach services and community linkage work. This is not surprising, as a new system must emerge out of the old. It is to be expected that vested interests within the old system will try to become players within the new if they cannot stop the change from taking place. The fact that the institutional sector is seeking to enter community care suggests such shifts are now inevitable.

Consistent with and integral to some community approaches is a life-style, health-promotion approach to care. This incorporates the concept of empowerment for seniors and for families. While the concept has become very popular, many of the issues in terms of whether this inevitably means disempowerment for health care workers have not been tackled in any systematic way. Implications of this approach for the entire health care system have not been debated. Indeed, the question is only starting to be asked.

The health care system in Canada is in a state of flux not seen for many decades. The new vision of an appropriate health care system for Canadians is exciting and holds much promise. It provides an opportunity for greater recognition of and participation by caregivers. At the same time, it holds the danger that the burden of care will be shifted more to their shoulders. We do not yet know the details of the system that will emerge but now is the time for families and caregivers to make their wishes known.

REFERENCES

Antonucci, T.C. (1990). Social supports and social relationships. In R.H. Binstock & L.K. George (Eds.), *Handbook of aging and the social sciences* (3rd ed.). New York, NY: Academic Press.

Baker, P.M. (1987). *A survey of the need for sheltered housing for the elderly in greater Victoria*. Paper presented at the annual meeting of the Canadian Association on Gerontology, Calgary, Alberta.

Baldock, J., & Evers, A. (1991). Innovations and care of the elderly: The front line of change for social welfare services. *Ageing International*, XVIII, 8-21.

Barer, M.L., & Stoddart, G.L. (1991). *Toward integrated medical resource policies for Canada: Background document*. Vancouver, BC: Health Policy Research Unit, Centre for Health Services and Policy Research, University of British Columbia.

Berliner, H.S. (1977). Emerging ideologies in medicine. *Review Radical Political Economics, 9*, 116-124.

Blendon, R.J. (1989). Three systems: A comparative survey. *Health Management Quarterly, 11*, 2-10.

Chambers, L.W., Labelle, R., Gafni, A., & Goeree, R. (1992). *The organization and financing of public and private sector long term care facilities for the elderly in Canada. Report on Part I: Survey of the provinces.* Working paper #92-13. Hamilton, ON: Centre for Health Economics and Policy Analysis, McMaster University.

Chappell, N.L. (1992). *Social support and aging.* Toronto, ON: Butterworths.

Doty, P. (1988). Long-term care in international perspective. *Health Care Financing Review*, Annual Supplement.

Estes, C.L., & Wood, J.B. (1986). The non-profit sector and community-based care for the elderly in the U.S.: A disappearing resource? *Social Science and Medicine, 23*, 1261-1266.

Evans, R.G., & Stoddart, G.L. (1990). Producing health, consuming health care. *Social Science & Medicine, 31*, 1347-1363.

General Accounting Office. (1991). *Canadian health insurance: Lessons for the United States.* Gaithersburg, MD: U.S. General Accounting Office.

George, L.K. (1988). *Why won't caregivers use community services? Unexpected findings from a respite care demonstration/evaluation.* Paper presented at the annual meeting of the Gerontological Society of America, San Francisco, California.

Gonyea, J.G. (1988). *Alzheimer's disease support groups: How do members benefit?* Paper presented at the annual meeting of the Gerontological Society of America, San Francisco, California.

Habitat. (1989). *Habitat: A national seniors housing consultation.* Ottawa, ON: One Voice–The Canadian Seniors Network.

Heagerty, B., Dunn, L., & Watson, M.A. (1988). Helping caregivers care. *Aging, 358*, 7-10.

Health and Welfare Canada. (1991). *Description of long-term care services in provinces and territories of Canada.* Ottawa, ON: Federal/Provincial/Territorial Subcommittee on Continuing Care, Health Services Directorate, Health Services and Promotion Branch.

Horowitz, A., Sherman, R.H., & Durmanskin, S.C. (1983). *Employment and daughter caregivers: A working partnership for older people?* Paper presented at the annual meeting of the Gerontological Society of America, San Francisco, California.

Kane, R.L., Evans, J.G., & Macfadyen, D. (Eds). (1990). *Improving the health of older people: A world view.* World Health Organization.

Lomas, J. (1990). Finding audiences, changing beliefs: The structure of research use in Canadian health policy. *Journal of Health Politics, Policy and Law, 15*, 525-542.

Lubben, J.E., Weiler, P.G., & Chi, I. (1989). Health practices of the elderly poor. *American Journal of Public Health, 79*, 731-34.

Manitoba Health. (1992). *Quality health for Manitobans: The action plan.* Winnipeg, MB: Partners for Health, Manitoba Health.

McPherson, K. (1990). International differences in medical care practices. In *Health care systems in transition: The search for efficiency* (OECD Social Policy Studies No. 7). Ottawa ON: Renouf Publishing Company Ltd.

Muldoon, J.M., & Stoddart, G.L. (1989). Publicly financed competition in health care delivery–a Canadian assimilation model. *Journal of Health Economics, 8*, 313-338.

National Council on Welfare. (1990). *Health, health care and medicare.* Ottawa, ON: Minister of Supply and Services Canada.

Noelker, L.S., & Poulshock, S.W. (1982). *The effects on families of caring for impaired elderly in residence.* Washington, DC: U.S. Department of Health and Human Services, Administration on Aging.

Porter, B. (1991). *The health care system in Canada and its funding: No easy solutions.* Ottawa, ON: Canada Communication Group-Publishing, Supply and Services Canada.

Province of British Columbia. (1991). *Closer to home: The report of the British Columbia royal commission on health care and costs.* Victoria, B.C.: Crown Publications Inc.

Rakowski, W., & Clark, N.M. (1985). Future outlook, caregiving, and care-receiving in the family context. *The Gerontologist, 25,* 618-623.

Saperstein, A.R. (1988). *Respite service: A service model.* Paper presented at the annual meeting of the Gerontological Society of America, San Francisco, California.

Scott, J.P., & Roberto, K.A. (1985). Use of informal and formal support networks by rural elderly poor. *The Gerontologist, 25,* 624-630.

Shapiro, E. (1991). *Manitoba health care studies and their policy implications.* Winnipeg, MB: Manitoba Centre for Health Policy and Evaluation, Department of Community Health Sciences, University of Manitoba.

Statistics Canada. (1988).

Social Policies Regarding Caregiving to Elders: Canadian Contradictions

Susan A. McDaniel, PhD

University of Alberta, Edmonton, Alberta, Canada

Ellen M. Gee, PhD

Simon Fraser University, Burnaby, British Columbia, Canada

SUMMARY. In Canada, disparate social policies–to do with health, family, income security, housing, and so forth–influence caregiving to elders. They are contradictory policies because of their different objectives, histories, and jurisdictions. The wider context of societal and socio-demographic changes highlight additional contradictions in the principles on which social policies regarding caregiving rest. Some of these contradictions are discussed in terms of policies, their consequences, whether intended or not, and what the future might hold for Canadian policies and programs with implications for caregiving to elders.

Susan A. McDaniel has been Professor of Sociology at University of Alberta since 1988. Her current research includes aging and social policy, the aging work force, and balancing work and family in mid-life. Ellen M. Gee is Professor of Sociology at Simon Fraser University. Her current research interests include aging families, women and aging, social policies related to aging, lone parent families, and age norms.

Address correspondence to: Susan A. McDaniel, Department of Sociology, University of Alberta, Edmonton, Alberta T6G 2H4, Canada.

[Haworth co-indexing entry note]: "Social Policies Regarding Caregiving to Elders: Canadian Contradictions," McDaniel, Susan A., and Ellen M. Gee. Co-published simultaneously in the *Journal of Aging & Social Policy*, (The Haworth Press, Inc.) Vol. 5, No. 1/2, 1993, pp. 57-72; and: *International Perspectives on State and Family Support for the Elderly* (ed: Scott A. Bass and Robert Morris) The Haworth Press, Inc., 1993, pp. 57-72. Multiple copies of this article/chapter may be purchased from The Haworth Document Delivery Center [1-800-3-HAWORTH; 9:00 a.m. - 5:00 p.m. (EST)].

57

Caregiving is being given a second look by social analysts in the 1990s. The impetus comes from two very different sources. On the one hand, caregiving, largely done by women whether for pay or out of family duty, is beginning to be examined as work (Aronson, 1990, 1991; Baines, Evans, & Neysmith, 1991; Chappell, 1989; Gee & McDaniel, 1992; Kaden & McDaniel, 1990; McDaniel, 1992b, 1992d; Neysmith, 1989). On the other hand, economic constraints, combined with a growing need for care, have made caregiving a public issue (Angus, 1991; Gee & McDaniel, 1992; Jutras, 1990; Lero et al., 1992; Matras, 1990; McDaniel, 1992c; Myles & Quadagno, 1991; Walker, 1991). The two approaches come together in "the caregiving crunch," as fewer women are available, or have time available, for the work required in caregiving (Myles, 1991, p. 82), at the same time as other options are being reduced. Thus, caregiving has been thrust firmly onto the stage of public policy debate and challenge.

Caregiving to elderly people is being acknowledged as one of the fundamental challenges facing Western societies (Jutras, 1990, p. 763). John Myles states unequivocally that "The next crisis of the welfare state will be a result of the 'care-giving crunch' and it is already with us" (Myles, 1991, p. 82). And yet, little analysis has been done in Canada of the caregiving implications, both intended and unintended, of existing social policies. This article aims to examine Canadian policies regarding caregiving to elders in a social context, focusing on their objectives, histories, jurisdictions, and, most centrally, the principles that underlie the policies. This article does not seek to be comprehensive, but rather focuses on contexts and contradictions relying on particular policies as illustrations.

CONTEXT/ANALYTICAL FRAMEWORK

Social policies with caregiving implications can be understood only in their context, not just the specific context in which the policies develop, but also the wider context of social and demographic change. Social policies in capitalist countries typically grow out of one or more of the following: a perceived need to redress inequities; to modify or lessen the play of market forces; to serve ideological or political purposes; or for other reasons related to political or economic exigencies. In the interest of space, only four contextual factors for caregiving will be discussed here, and those only briefly.

Demographic aging poses challenges to social policy on caregiving, not because it necessarily produces a crisis for the public purse as some analysts and many politicians have argued, but rather because it occurs in the context of family changes, value adjustments, changes in causes of death, and gender differentials in life expectancy. In demographically older societies, families tend to have smaller numbers of children and greater numbers of generations, and there is a greater disparity among generation sizes. More people die of chronic illnesses and late in life, and women tend to outlive men. Demographically aged societies have high standards of living, with expectations that health care and essential social needs will be met by one means or another.

In Canada, there is recognition in policy circles that demographic aging results from low birth rates. Policy responses to this have ranged from Quebec's policy of increasing baby bonus payments to families with increasing birth orders, to discussion at the federal level of raising immigration levels to compensate partially for the low birth rates among Canadians (Gee & McDaniel, 1992). Although immigration levels are not likely to be raised sufficiently to counter Canada's low birth rate, Canada's active immigration policy and policies of multiculturalism have meant that Canada is a mix of ethnic groups, with many recent immigrants. The Canadian multi-ethnic population has important implications for caregiving.

The twin pillars of *markets and politics* have been, and continue to be, more important to the development and maintenance of social policies in Canada than in other Western capitalist countries. The reason is that Canada's income-security policies and programs are essentially dualistic, at once modifying the impact of market forces on the elderly, while at the same time, allowing the market within the limits of government supports to play out on the rest of the population (Myles & Quadagno, 1991, p. 86).

Only in the late 1980s and 1990s has the rhetoric of deficit begun to be the guiding paradigm of governments, both federal and provincial, in Canada. It is deficit as paradigm that is behind the undermining of universality for popular programs such as Old Age Security, as the payments are "clawed back" by income taxes, without being indexed. The claw-back affects seniors with incomes above $50,000 (Canadian) in the first year, but gradually cuts deeper and deeper into the incomes of seniors, in effect producing a benefit that is universal in name only (Gee & McDaniel, 1991).

No one can have missed the *growing centrality of family to the political agenda* in the 1990s, both in the United States and in Canada. In the United States, there was Vice-President Quayle with his notion that a television character, Murphy Brown, was responsible for the surmised decline in "family values" in her decision to have a child outside of marriage. In Canada, there is the "Family Caucus," a group of influential members of the Progressive Conservative party who serve as Members of Parliament and work to resist changes in social policy that might be detrimental to "traditional family values," such as day care programs, women's rights in the workplace, or the granting of equal rights to gays and lesbians. Although given less press, this Caucus is also concerned about families "abandoning" their elderly, despite the evidence that few Canadians are institutionalized, and the majority of those are the very frail, very old elderly.

A recurrent theme in the political and policy concerns about families is the importance of families for society. An aspect of this preoccupation is the assumption that family care is the best kind of care for children as well as for elders. The focus has been almost exclusively on the beneficiary of family care rather than on the caregiver (Aronson, 1991; Chappell, 1989; McDaniel, 1992d; 1992e; Neysmith, 1989).

The *women's movement and growing awareness of women's issues* provides another context for social policies concerned with caregiving in Canada (Gee & Kimball, 1987). Feminist research has made clear that what is done at home by women for no remuneration is work that benefits families and societies in accountable ways. Research by feminists has also shown that caregiving work may be coerced from women by defining a "good" woman as one who cares for others ahead of herself (Aronson, 1990). Marge

Reitsma-Street (1991) reveals that women who do not sufficiently accept the notion that caring for others is the way women should construct their lives and identities are penalized socially and even legally (in the case of adolescent delinquents). Political feminists, through lobbying efforts and research, have put the issues of women's unpaid work as caregivers to the young, the old, spouses, the sick, and the disabled on the political agenda (Baines, Evans & Neysmith, 1991; Lero et al., 1992; McDaniel, 1992a; 1992d). Women's issues have become important in the political process. And Canadian women, unlike their sisters in the United States, have achieved constitutional acknowledgement of equal rights.

In a rudimentary sense, a framework for the analysis of caregiving policies might include the following: consideration of caregiving as work, valuable work that benefits society; exploration of the links between caregiving work and labor markets; attention to the gender inequities of caregiving as currently structured, with exploration of the implications; examination of the assumptions of family care (is it always desirable? wanted? congruent with the interests of elders?); consideration that caregiving might be reciprocal; exploration of the assumptions about congruency between family and household, and what this means regarding the presumptions of caregiver availability; attention to the public responsibility for caregiving to elders and any potential costs of not taking that responsibility; and examination of the ways in which responsibility for caregiving to elders is shared by society, families, and elders themselves.

CANADIAN POLICIES ON CAREGIVING

The Canadian welfare state is structured around the needs of a "young" population. Even the policies of major importance to older persons–income security and health–were implemented with aims other than serving the aged. For example, Canadian national health insurance (established in 1968) is dominated by a medical model geared to the health needs of younger people; further, its implementation was supported by business interests, which saw socialized medicine as a way to pass on to taxpayers the costs of ensuring a healthy labor force (Lightman & Irving, 1991). Similarly, the Old Age Security Act of 1951 (preceded by the Old Age

Pensions Act of 1927) and the Canada Pension Plan (CPP) of 1968 were aimed as much at inducing older people out of the labor force–in order to make room for younger, less expensive workers–as at providing an adequate income for the aged (McDonald & Wanner, 1990). (Indeed, the large numbers of poor aged made necessary the implementation of need-based programs–the Guaranteed Income Supplement [implemented in 1975], and provincial income supplements, commencing in 1972 in British Columbia.) In a related vein, the Federal Supreme Court in 1991 upheld mandatory retirement at age 65, arguing that such age-based discrimination benefitted the "common good" (i.e., maximized the employment chances of younger people). Rhetoric aside, Canadian public policy has not adjusted to a changing age structure.

Policy is linked to Canadian federalism, the relationship between the Dominion and the provinces. The British North America Act of 1867 gave the federal government jurisdiction over important social and economic matters, and left to the provinces responsibilities of a minor nature–as perceived at the time. What we now think of as "health and welfare" was deemed minor (by default, as this was not mentioned in the BNA Act) and thus, the responsibility of the provinces. As society changed and "health and welfare" took on increasing importance, the provinces had the responsibility but not the finances to cope. As a result, an uneasy liaison between the federal and provincial governments developed. The federal government did not have the "right"; the provincial government did not have the money. Provincial responsibility for welfare, upheld in the patriated Constitution of 1982, has led to a complex and uncoordinated system with provincial differences in service availability, standards (including access criteria), and funding.

As a result of these particular characteristics of the Canadian welfare state–a tendency to favor the young and lack of coordination–policies concerning the aged and caregiving have developed in an ad hoc fashion and are fraught with internal contradictions. (See Table 1 for an overview of policies related to elder caregiving.)

Four examples of such contradictions are provided here. One, the medical, physician-oriented, and cure-based nature of the health system is unsuited to older persons, who typically have chronic conditions with social dimensions. This lack of fit results in health

Table 1: Major Canadian Social Policies/Programs with Caregiving
        Implications

Policy Area	Major Policies/ Programs	Jurisdiction	Criteria
Health	•Medicare	•provinces (cost-sharing)*	•universal
	•Long-term care	•provinces (various)**	•health status (some programs need-based)
Income	•OAS	•federal	•universal (but claw-back)
	•CPP***	•federal	•contributory
	•GIS/SPA	•federal	•need
	•supplements	•some provinces	•need
	•Private pensions	•federal/ provincial/ employer	•workplace-dependent
	•RRSPs	•federal	•"merit"
Social Services	•Home support	•provincial -with federal and municipal (cost-sharing)*	•need
	•Rehabilitation	-as above	•need
	•Retirement homes	-as above	•need
Housing	•Core housing need	•federal and provinces (various)**	•need
	•Property tax rebate	•provinces	•age (and home ownership)
	•Housing allowance	•provinces (some)	•need
Workplace	•Eldercare assistance	•employer	•workplace-dependent
	•Mandatory retirement	•federal/ provincial	•age

*with federal government
**various funding arrangements between federal and provincial
     governments
*** province of Quebec administers own plan

care that is expensive and not particularly effective for old people.
(It also creates a convenient scapegoat–the aging of the population–
for rising health care costs.) Increasing costs, in conjunction with
reductions in federal transfer payments, have led to the real possibility that universalistic health care in Canada will be abandoned,

bringing with it the risk that the health needs of substantial numbers of poorer elderly persons will be neglected altogether. In the long run, this would have very costly implications.

Two, the discrepancies in availability and accessibility associated with an uncoordinated system can be seen with regard to respite care, the most needed service from the point of view of "hands-on" caregivers (Chappell, 1989). In some places, respite care is provided under provincial government long-term care policy; in others, it is available only from for-profit organizations for persons willing and/or able to pay. Thus, the availability of a crucial service vis-à-vis caregiving varies, depending on provincial-federal "deals."

Three, policies and programs in Canada have been geared to aged persons as individuals. However, caregiving involves a caregiver and a care recipient, who might require assistance from different policy arenas, and each of whom might or might not be eligible for programs (National Advisory Council on Aging, 1990), depending on their characteristics and where they live. For example, respite care involves resources from both health and social services–this puts an additional demand for coordination on a policy and delivery system already plagued with such problems. Another example is from the housing policy area, in which the need criterion discourages co-residence of the caregiver and the recipient when one or the other is not categorized as "low income" by government definitions. (This is an important mechanism for encouraging independent living, as long as proper supports are in place.)

Four, reforms are blocked or delayed due to the required–and delicate–negotiations between the federal and provincial governments built into the Canadian system. One reform is a "drop-out" provision in the CPP, which would allow caregivers to exit from paid employment for a period of time in order to attend to caregiving duties without losing pension credits. (There is such a provision in the CPP for child care.) Our recent history illustrates that provincial opposition to CPP reform can be effective and divisive (a proposal to increase benefits was vetoed by Ontario and eventually defeated, during what was called the Great Pension Debate [late 1970s]). Thus, attempts to launch the CPP drop-out provision for elder caregivers require strong federal support and provincial consensus. In the meantime, caregivers run the risk of "burn-out," and care recipients who lose their primary caregiver are at risk of institutional placement.

We have seen that internal contradictions regarding caregiving result from the overall nature of the Canadian welfare state. Next, we turn to caregiving policy contradictions stemming from broader aspects of Canadian society and of Western capitalist societies.

CAREGIVING POLICY CONTRADICTIONS

In Canada, from the end of the Second World War until the 1970s, a Keynesian welfare state was erected, with a distinct Canadian style (McDaniel & Agger, 1982). The very beginnings of the welfare state in Canada were focused on issues of old age, not in the interest of "serving" the elderly, but to benefit the labor market and the economy. Unlike in the United States and United Kingdom, where the "crisis of the welfare state" has become a rallying cry, in Canada the issues of the welfare state have centered largely on pensions and how best to expand, not contract, them. Discussions of generational inequities, so prevalent in the United States, have received virtually no attention north of the 49th parallel (Gee & McDaniel, 1992; Osberg, 1991).

Canadian social policy has grown out of a number of uneasy contradictions and compromises. The universalistic health care system in Canada, for example, is both accessible to all and protective of the interest of business. Public pensions grew out of much the same contradiction–to ease expensive workers out of the work force with some degree of dignity, but to make room for less expensive and less demanding, younger workers. As John Myles and Jill Quadagno (1991) have shown, no sooner was the first public pension scheme in place in Canada but it was contentious. The tension between public pensions as social welfare and as support to the labor market was clear in Canada from the outset.

It is, in part, the rich social policy network in Canada that makes for contradictions. As shown in Table 1, jurisdictional responsibilities for the various policies and programs with caregiving implications range from federal to provincial (with some municipalities involved in housing and social services, for example) and from public to private. This means, minimally, that policies and programs get caught in wrangling about who is responsible for what and, as the Canadian institution of transfer payments between governments shows, to what degree they are responsible. Social policies in Canada have become part of economic policy (most visibly in the recent free trade negotiations, first with the United States and then with Mexico and the United States) as some trading partners suggest that Canadian social programs subsidized certain goods and services. The public vs. private dilemma has been a recurring theme with Canadian social policies as well. The issue of affordability of Canada's "safety net" programs and policies has been raised by politicians with increasing frequency, for example. Recently, there has been a clear move toward privatization of a variety of social programs, particularly those related to caregiving such as home care, visitation of nurses, meal delivery, and so forth, and to encouraging the private sector to do more in terms of workplace policies with social benefits.

The income maintenance/generational transfer scheme in Canada, including but not limited to pensions of the various sorts listed in Table 1, provides an illustration of some of the more daunting contradictions in Canadian social policy on caregiving. In principle, pensions provide income for the nonworking by monies provided by the working, so there is a generational transfer of wealth. In the Canadian case, there is the presumption additionally that public pensions will not only supplement private pensions, but that the policy of public pensions will be an inducement to the development of private plans (which has not happened). Further, there is the implicit assumption that there will be generational transfers, from old to young and from young to old within families. All of these income transfers presume stability of generational size and family structure (Osberg, 1991). Yet, this is not the case at all in Canada. Demographic aging has meant that larger and less well off generations follow smaller, better off generations, and where family changes have meant that baby boomers, when facing old age, will have not only a smaller pool of family caregivers to whom to turn as a result of lower birth rates and family dissolution but also less asset accumulation than their parents' generation. Asset accumulation may be particularly problematic for the growing numbers of single mothers with children. As well, many of those who retire with the baby-boom generation may have had capital flows and caregiving responsibilities outside of Canada, as they support relatives elsewhere. The tripartite presumption of public, private, and familial generational income transfers may not work in the future, and likely has not worked well in the past.

Canadian policies of caregiving to elders, for the most part, have assumed that family care and support are given. It is widely thought that social policies on caregiving start where family care ends, either in a crisis situation, when a family caregiver is unavailable, or when support for the family caregiver is needed. An alternative argument, gaining support as evidence accumulates, is that elders and their families suffer *as a consequence* of existing social policies on caregiving (Jutras, 1990; McDaniel, 1990, 1992c, 1991d; Neysmith, 1989, p. 141). Stated in its most simple terms, this argument holds that social policies on caregiving by reinforcing traditional family structures, values, and authorities both in the family and the state make women, who comprise the vast majority of caregivers, vulnerable to policies that define them as essentially familial. Home care policy in Canada, which argues that the goal must be to keep elders in their homes as long as possible, would be but one example of placing extreme burden and responsibility on wives, daughters, and daughters-in-law.

The increasing subordination of social policy to economic policy has meant that the "residual" perspective, whereby the "free" market metes out justice and resources to individuals on the basis of need, takes priority over the institutional perspective of providing benefits universally. What this perspective overlooks are the economic benefits accorded to society *by* social programs. One example, the much beleaguered Canadian public health care insurance program, has been labeled as too expensive to remain universal, yet when General Motors cited financial difficulties in its recent plant closings in the United States, one of the most expensive items mentioned was the cost of private health insurance for its employees, a cost much higher than it is for General Motors employees in Canada. With respect to caregiving, the interests of economic policy and Canada have modified the basis on which benefits are allocated, from entitlement to merit, or need (Matras, 1990). Increasingly then, both the elder and the caregiver are subject to the forces of the market, in an unbuffered way. And yet caregiving is seen by policy as nonmarket activity.

The rapidly changing relationship between the family and the state reveals additional aspects of contradiction in Canadian policies on caregiving. As Alan Walker (1991, pp. 95-96) argues, the compelling failure is of the state to meet either the needs of the caregiver or those of the elder; in the process, a wedge is driven between the two. The essential problem is the ideology of familism by which social policies see families as they never were, and certainly with today's rapid socio-demographic and economic changes, as they never can be (Bane & Jargowsky, 1988; Eichler, 1987; Jenson, 1989; Kaden & McDaniel, 1990; McDaniel, 1989, 1990, 1992b). Caregiving by "families," a euphemism for *women* in families, is so presumed that the dwindling numbers of women available for work, and the lack of support they face, is invisible to social policies on caregiving. The myth of families abandoning their elders and of women not doing enough caregiving prevails over the reality that most of it is still provided within a family context, with the caregiver absorbing the shocks of the changing family and context in which the care is provided. The strong endorsements that policies relating to community and home care in Canada have received suggest that future policies will encourage the unpaid labor of women at home to care for elders as a substitute for formal health or social services, with no serious consideration of the caregiver whose work is thought to fall beyond the bounds of the market.

TOWARD AN AMBIGUOUS FUTURE

The shape of the future is written in the present and the past, so to that extent the contradictions and tensions of policies of today and yesterday are likely to shape the policies of the future. Rather than attempt to predict the future, our purpose here is to adopt the concept of analytical credibility, which focuses on how to use research in decisionmaking, and on creating rather than discovering the future.

What do we know about social policies on caregiving in Canada? In sum, we know that demand for caregiving is likely to increase in the future and that existing policies are largely inadequate to meet that need. We know that existing policies are a hodgepodge, designed for other purposes and other times, only partially meeting the needs of elders and generally failing caregivers in substantial ways. We know that social policies are asking families to do more and more at the same time that women in families have evermore limited time and energy for all the demands placed on them. And we know that the contradictions on which policies regarding caregiving rest will become more and more sharp, with some possibly destroying the effectiveness (such as it is) of existing policies. More important than what is known from research is the inattentiveness of policymaking in Canada, for the most part, to what research produces in regard to caregiving and caregiving policies.

Perhaps most important is not what is known about policies regarding caregiving, but what remains to be known. More theoretical understanding is needed about how social policy and societal structures actually play out in people's lives to shape their experiences of caregiving and care receiving. In particular, more needs to be known about how caregiving shapes women's lives, opportunities, aspirations, and old age. The costs and benefits–both in terms of dollars and lost opportunities–of caregiving for no pay or for pay should be examined and weighed. In Nova Scotia, the only province that provides remuneration to caregivers, the evidence is that stresses felt by caregivers continue. Similarly, the costs and benefits of universal programs versus targeting should be explored. The ways in which caregiving at home is mirrored in the workplace, particularly among women, needs exploration. The unspoken assumptions of caregiving policies should be examined, such as: the presumption that familial caregiving is a solution to a problem, rather than a problem in itself; that it should be given and is to be expected by social policy; that it is desired by elders; that it is provided voluntarily and out of love; that it will not result in abuse and neglect of the elder or of the caregiver herself, by her family and, indeed, by social policies that force her into the caregiving role. Just as child care has served as a catalyst that has revealed much about family, gender, and work and how they interconnect, so could caregiving to elders.

The ways in which the knowledge base about caregiving and social policy are or are not considered in the building of future policies will determine, in part, what kind of future is created. Research that explores the costs and benefits of caregiving policies might well show that support of caregivers has benefits that include cost-savings as well as the increased likelihood of both elders and caregivers living into old age in a healthy state. The history and infrastructure of Canada's social policies makes the country an ideal place to develop explicit caregiving policies that could dovetail, for example, with proposed changes in the health care system, making it less medically based, and more health care oriented. Yet, caution must be exercised in any undertaking to rationalize Canadian social policies on caregiving that could deprive Canadians of the strengths that the history of contradictory policies has provided, a strength that builds on something more than market forces.

In 1993, it is difficult to muster much optimism about the future of caregiving policies in Canada. A national referendum on a new constitutional agreement, the Charlottetown Accord, was soundly defeated in October 1992. While the new Constitution would have further decentralized powers from the federal government to the provinces, its defeat is not without challenges to social policy in Canada. Further discussions and negotiations on constitutional matters have been "laid to rest" for the foreseeable future, but cannot be neglected forever, given the precarious constitutional situation of Quebec, which never signed the Constitution when it was repatriated to Canada in 1982. A continuation of the hodgepodge of Canadian social policies on caregiving seems assured.

AUTHOR NOTE

Susan A. McDaniel previously was on the faculty at the University of Waterloo for 13 years. She is the author of two books and more than 100 publications in the areas of aging, family, gender and demography. Her book "Aging and Policy in Canada" (with Ellen Gee) is now being completed. Ellen M. Gee is the author of more than 50 publications in the areas of aging, family, and demography.

REFERENCES

Angus, D. (1991). *Caring communities: Highlights of the symposium on social supports*. Ottawa: Statistics Canada.

Aronson, J. (1990). Older women's experience needing care: Choice or compulsion. *Canadian Journal on Aging, 9* (3), 234-247.

Aronson, J. (1991). Dutiful daughters and undemanding mothers: Contrasting images of giving and receiving care in middle and later life. In C. Baines, P. Evans & S. Neysmith (Eds.), *Women's caring: Feminist perspectives on social welfare* (pp. 138-168). Toronto: McClelland and Stewart.

Baines, C., Evans, P. & Neysmith, S. (Eds.). (1991). *Women's caring: Feminist perspectives on social welfare*. Toronto: McClelland and Stewart.

Chappell, N. (1989). *Formal programs for informal caregivers to elders*. Report to the Aging Policy Section, Health Policy Division, Ottawa: Health and Welfare Canada.

Eichler, M. (1987). Family change and social policies. In K. Anderson, H. Armstrong, P. Armstrong, J. Drackich et al., (Eds.), *Family matters* (pp. 63-85). Toronto: Methuen.

Gee, E.M., & Kimball, M. (1987). *Women and aging*. Toronto: Butterworths.

Gee, E.M., & McDaniel, S.A. (1991). Pension politics and challenges: Retirement policy implications. *Canadian Public Policy, 27* (4), 456-472.

Gee, E.M., & McDaniel, S.A. (1992). Social policy for an aging Canada. *Journal of Canadian Studies, 27* (3).

Jenson, A.M. (1989). Caregiving and socialization in view of declining fertility and increasing female employment. *Marriage & Family Review, 14* (1/2), 127-144.

Jutras, S. (1990). Caring for the elderly: The partnership issue. *Social Sciences and Medicine, 31* (7), 763-771.

Kaden, J., & McDaniel, S.A. (1990). Caregiving and care-receiving: A double bind for women in Canada's aging society. *Journal of Women and Aging, 2* (3), 3-26.

Lero, D.C., Pense, A.R., Shields, M., Brockman, L.M., & Goelman, H. (1992). *Canadian national child care study: Introductory report*. Ottawa: Statistics Canada. Cata. No. 89-526E.

Lightman, E., & Irving, A. (1991). Restructuring Canada's welfare state. *Journal of Social Policy, 20*, 65-86.

Matras, J. (1990). *Dependency, obligations and entitlements: A new sociology of aging, the life course and the elderly*. Englewood Cliffs, New Jersey: Prentice Hall.

McDaniel, S.A. (1989). Women and aging: A sociological perspective. *Journal of Women and Aging, 1* (1-3), 47-67.

McDaniel, S.A. (1990). Towards family policy in Canada with women in mind. *Feminist Perspectives* (Canadian Research Institute for the Advancement of Women), *17*, 1-32.

McDaniel, S.A. (1992a). Women and family in the later years: Findings from the 1990 General Social Survey. *Canadian Woman Studies, 12* (2), 62-64.

McDaniel, S.A. (1992b). *Life rhythms and caring: Aging, family and the state.* Saskatoon, Saskatchewan: University of Saskatchewan, Sorokin Series.

McDaniel, S.A. (1992c). Families, feminism and the state. In L. Samuelson & B. Marshall (Eds), *Social problems: Thinking critically.* Toronto: Garamond.

McDaniel, S.A. (1992d). Caring and sharing: Demographic aging, family and the state. In J. Hendricks & C. Rosenthal (Eds.). *The remainder of their days: Impact of public policy on older families.* New York: Garland Press.

McDaniel, S.A. (1992e, June 2). *Women and older Canadians in families: The caring crunch.* Paper presented at a joint session of the Canadian Population Society and the Canadian Association of Sociology and Anthropology meetings, Charlottetown, Prince Edward Island.

McDaniel, S.A., & Agger, B. (1982). *Social problems through conflict and order.* Don Mills, Ontario: Addison-Wesley.

McDonald, P.L., & Wanner, R.A. (1990). *Retirement in Canada.* Toronto: Butterworths.

Myles, J. (1991). Editorial: Women, the welfare state and caregiving. *Canadian Journal on Aging, 10* (2), 82-85.

Myles, J., & Quadagno, J. (Eds). (1991). *States, labor markets and the future of old-age policy.* Philadelphia: Temple University Press.

National Advisory Council on Aging. (1990). *The NACA position on informal caregiving: Support and enhancement.* Ottawa: Minister of Supply and Services.

Neysmith, S. (1989). Closing the gap between health policy and the home-care needs of tomorrow's elderly. *Canadian Journal of Community Mental Health, 8* (2), 141-150.

Osberg, L. (1991). *Inequality between generations and the role of the family.* Report prepared for the Demographic Review, Health and Welfare Canada.

Reitsma-Street, M. (1991). Girls learn to care; Girls policed to care. In C. Baines, P. Evans, and S. Neysmith (Eds.), *Women's caring: Feminist perspectives on social welfare* (pp. 106-137). Toronto: McClelland and Stewart.

Walker, A. (1991). The relationship between the family and the state in the care of older people. *Canadian Journal on Aging, 10* (2), 94-112.

Paid Family Caregiving:
A Review of Progress and Policies

Lynn B. Gerald, MA

University of South Alabama
Mobile, Alabama

SUMMARY. Policymakers in the United States have begun to examine solutions that encourage increased sharing of caregiving responsibilities between government and family. Initiatives in Sweden and the United Kingdom are now in place. Support includes a care leave policy implemented at the federal level, paying salaries to family members when caregiving is a regular job, providing job training to salaried caregivers when their personal caregiving experience ends, community-based programs for caregivers, and allowances to be used for providing care to an elderly person.

In the United States, 13 states pay caregivers as Medicaid providers. Policymakers have considered tax incentives and, in 1975, U.S. Senate Bill 1161 was introduced but failed as an attempt to provide cash subsidies to families caring for the elderly. A proposal has been made to expand the Temporary Disability Model to include care of family members of all ages by providing adequate wage replacement

---

Lynn B. Gerald is Research Associate in the Department of Sociology and Anthropology at the University of South Alabama. Her research interests are in family-care policies and physical fitness.

The author wishes to express her appreciation for review and comments by Dr. Roma Hanks, University of South Alabama, Department of Sociology and Anthropology, and Dr. Konrad Kressley, University of South Alabama, Department of Political Science.

[Haworth co-indexing entry note]: "Paid Family Caregiving: A Review of Progress and Policies," Gerald, Lynn B. Co-published simultaneously in the *Journal of Aging & Social Policy,* (The Haworth Press, Inc.) Vol. 5, No. 1/2, 1993, pp. 73-89; and: *International Perspectives on State and Family Support for the Elderly* (ed: Scott A. Bass and Robert Morris) The Haworth Press, Inc., 1993, pp. 73-89. Multiple copies of this article/chapter may be purchased from The Haworth Document Delivery Center [1-800-3-HAWORTH; 9:00 a.m. - 5:00 p.m. (EST)].

73

to assist caregivers. At present, 34 states provide some type of economic support for caregivers. Research is needed to determine what types of programs are most acceptable and beneficial to caregivers as well as cost effective for government.

A dramatic increase in life expectancy in the United States has taken place from the years 1900 to 1992. In 1900, the average life expectancy at birth for a male was 46 years and for a female it was 49 years. Now, life expectancy is about 72 years for males and 79 years for females (Social Security Administration, 1989). This increase in life expectancy coupled with other social and demographic trends such as lower birth rates and technological advances in medicine has led to a great increase in the elderly population. In the years between 1915 and 1990, the birth rate dropped from 25 births per 1,000 persons to 14.9 births. Projections suggest that the birth rate will continue to decline, reaching 13.5 in 1995 and 12.6 in the year 2000 (U.S. Bureau of the Census, 1990). An exception to the decrease in birth rates occurred during the years 1946 to 1964. During this period, some 76 million Americans were born, creating what is now commonly known as the "baby boom" (Pifer & Bronte, 1986). This greatly affects dependency ratios (dependent young and older persons to the number of working persons). As the number of older persons continues to increase disproportionally in relation to the number of working persons, there will be growing problems of how to support our growing elderly population.

In addition to the increased number of elderly, there has been a rapid increase in the "oldest old," or those 85 years and older. The Social Security Administration (1984) has predicted that the 85-and-older population will more than double from 2,393,000 in 1980 to 5,161,000 in the year 2000. The great increase in this population is of concern because this is the population most likely to be in need of both medical and nonmedical help from a range of formal and informal sources (Manton, 1986). The living arrangements of this group also point out their high level of need. In 1980, 23.2% of those 85 and older lived in institutions (Rosenwaike, 1985). M. Barberis (1981) has observed that many people are placed in institutions to receive nonmedical assistance that could be provided at home. Estimates show that institutionalization could be prevented in 16% to 35% of these elderly if they received family and community support (Barberis, 1985). For this reason, policies regarding paid family care are important at this time.

Because of the increased number of older people, especially vulnerable elderly, there exists a large number of spouses and children who find themselves filling the caregiver role. Research has shown that caregivers have high depression rates, decreased life satisfaction, and feelings of anxiety, hopelessness, exhaustion, isolation, guilt, and anger (Brody, 1985; Cantor, 1983; Deimling & Bass, 1986; Fengler & Goodrich, 1979; George & Gwyther, 1986; Gilhooly, 1984; Haley, Levine, Brown, & Bartolucci, 1987; Haley, Levine, Brown, Berry, & Hughes, 1987; Jones & Vetter, 1984; Morycz, 1985; Rabins, Mace, & Lucas, 1982; Robinson & Thurnher, 1979; Sheehan & Nuttall, 1988).

In spite of high stress associated with caregiving, almost 80% of care to the elderly is provided by family members. Most caregivers are adult offspring, or spouses (Cantor, 1983). It is now estimated that about 72% of caregivers to the elderly are women (Stone, 1987; U.S. House of Representatives, 1987). They hold the social role of caregiver while also feeling the need for an income and a career. There is reason for concern for women of this "sandwich generation," who have the multiple responsibilities of mother, wife, and caregiver to an aging parent (Brody, 1981; Hooyman & Lustbader, 1986). David Biegel and Arthur Blum (1990) point out that the combination of decreased birth rates and increasing life expectancy is leading to a reversal in traditional caregiving patterns. According to the U.S. House Select Committee on Aging (1987), the average woman now spends 18 years of her life helping an elderly parent as compared to 17 years of her adult life caring for a dependent child. Traditionally, elder care was provided by women family members who were not employed outside the home. In 1950, only 36% of women between the ages of 25 and 54 worked. Today, the rate is 73% and is expected to rise to 80% by 1995 (Coberly, 1991). In addition, nursing home care is not available to most families because of the extreme costs. The average cost of a nursing home is about $25,000 to $30,000 per year at the present time and this is not covered under Medicare (*USA Today,* 1992). These costs are expected to rise as the need for nursing care and the population of the oldest old continues to grow. These factors all create great stress for these women caregivers.

Another confounding fact is that many of these adult children live separately from their parents and therefore the caregiver must spend time in maintaining two separate households. Because of the declining birth rate, there are now fewer children and siblings to share the responsibility for a parent's care. This places a larger burden on one person and creates many major life adjustments. As reported by caregivers, they are, for example:

> decreased free time for oneself, and decreased opportunities to socialize with one's friends, take vacations, have leisure time pursuits and run one's own house . . . Most caregivers protect their families and work, but at considerable personal expense to themselves. (Cantor, 1983, p. 600-601)

Research has shown that caregiving is emotionally and financially demanding of the caregiver. These factors combined often lead to the institutionalization of the elderly person (Krause et al., 1976; Morycz, 1985; Ross & Kedward, 1977; Tobin & Kulys, 1981). The burden of caregiving affects the quality of the caregiver's and the elder's lives and also has potential impact on the job performance of the caregiver, the number of elderly committed to nursing facilities and abuse of the elderly (Coberly, 1991; Kosberg, 1988; Neal, Chapman, Ingersoll-Dayton, Emlen, & Boise, 1990; Pearlman & Crown, 1992; Wagner, Creedon, Sasala, & Neal, 1989; Zarit, Reever, & Bach-Peterson, 1980).

A HISTORICAL PERSPECTIVE ON PAID CAREGIVING

Historically, there has been little formal financial support for long-term care services provided by the family. In fact, family members are often penalized for providing care because services and income benefits from Medicaid and Supplemental Security Insurance (SSI) are withheld from the elder when the family is providing care (Burwell, 1986). Demographic trends to do with longer lives and the increasing numbers of women working have brought forward concerns about costs to the government for the long-term care needs of the elderly. Policymakers have been forced to give attention to the development of long-term care policies that can meet the demand for services in the most economic and efficient manner. As this demand continues to grow, policymakers have a strong interest in maintaining the strength and durability of the informal caregiving network as the primary provider of long-term care services. They are interested in reducing the burden of caregivers but must also be concerned with additional costs to the government. A major goal of most economic initiatives is to reduce costs to the state by preventing the premature or unnecessary institutionalization of dependent elders.

Policymakers are also concerned with controlling the demand for caregiving compensation. Suzanne England (Osterbusch) and her associates (1990) point out two possible concerns about programs that pay caregivers. First, the "substitution effect" suggests that government compensation for caregivers will pay for care normally provided without compensation. Second, the "woodwork effect" proposes that the demand would overwhelm the system, meaning that individuals who are not receiving payment would ask for these benefits.

In studies of attitudes among agency personnel, researchers have investigated the advantages and disadvantages of implementing a paid family caregiving program (England et al., 1990, 1989; Simon-Rusinowitz, 1987). Only two advantages to paying family caregivers were listed by the agencies; this would (1) aid in providing continuity of care in that only one person would be responsible and workers would be available immediately to prevent lag time between need and placement of a worker and it would (2) increase the labor pool from which caregivers could be recruited, especially in areas where home health care is difficult to find.

The agencies cited many more disadvantages. These included the following: (1) assuring the quality of care and (2) dealing with general administration and payroll as well as problems of clients who have complaints about their care. England and her associates concluded that:

> the predominant agency view is that paid family members are qualitatively different from nonkin staff: They are different

and more difficult to train, to supervise, and to evaluate, and they are different to compensate. (1990, p. 81)

Issues around paid family caregiving are complex. The perspectives of family members, care receivers, and social service providers need to be heard if effective programs are to be put in place.

Greg Arling and William McAuley (1983) suggest several issues that must be considered by policymakers when devising a financial payment system for caregivers. The number of individuals who require daily living assistance is high and a financial payment system would have to limit payments to certain types of individuals if major costs are to be avoided. It is important to note that nonfinancial factors are often the greatest stressors faced by caregivers and that a financial payment system cannot relieve these pressures (Arling & McAuley, 1983). Financial payments have not been systematically proven as an effective method of motivating family care and this method has not been compared with others encouraging family care. Also, because informal care often comes from many sources, it is often hard to identify a primary caregiver. If only one person is chosen to receive compensation, others might feel that they were no longer needed or were not being sufficiently motivated. Research on specific caregiving arrangements and their contextual relationships is essential to the development of quality programs.

CROSS-CULTURAL PERSPECTIVES

We now shift our focus to some initiatives for paid family caregiving in Western Europe–specifically, Sweden and the United Kingdom–that could be used as models in building U.S. policy (Grana, 1983; Hokenstad & Johansson, 1990a, 1990b; Keigher, 1991). The new eldercare policy implemented in Sweden by the 1990 Care for the Elderly Bill reflects that society's concern for and commitment to family caregiving. Informal care is the largest source of support for older people in Sweden despite the fact that 80% of Swedish women 16 to 64 years of age are working (Hokenstad & Johansson, 1990b). The Swedish have already implemented at a federal level a care leave policy. Other supports that were to be enacted in 1992 include paying caregiver salaries to family members when caregiving is a regular job, providing labor market training to salaried caregivers when their personal caregiving experience ends, and service support policies that call for more community-based outreach programs to provide services to caregivers and help alleviate their burdens.

The care leave policy entitles persons to take time off from work and be paid an insurance allowance for up to 30 days to care for an elderly family member. A written application along with a doctor's statement of need for care is required to receive care leave benefits. Obviously, since the paid leave is limited to 30 days in the lifetime of the individual receiving the care, this is not meant to be used for ongoing caregiving situations but for the more acute illnesses.

The caregiver salaries are available to relatives of elders who provide at least 20 hours of care each week. These salaries are equivalent to those paid by home health care agencies and are provided by the government as taxable income with benefits including vacations and pensions. Merl Hokenstad and Lennarth Johansson (1990) found that there were more than 10,000 salaried family caregivers in Sweden. The government also encourages cities to provide labor market training for salaried caregivers when there is no longer a need for their paid family caregiving. The service supports such as respite care and homemaker services are very important to the caregivers in diminishing their stresses. The Swedish policy is probably the most comprehensive family caregiving support program in the world. It is likely to encourage family caregiving and make interaction easier between formal and informal caregiving services.

Another program not quite as comprehensive is one found in the United Kingdom (UK). Referred to as the Invalid Care Allowance (ICA), the UK program takes the form a regular allowance for providing care to a disabled or elderly person, who is separately entitled to an Attendance Allowance. The Attendance Allowance is a universal entitlement program to which any qualified disabled person has a right, regardless of income. This allowance is paid directly to the care receiver who may or may not choose to use it to purchase care. But, if a care receiver does get this allowance, their caregiver can apply for a separate ICA. Caregivers must be pre-retirement age to receive this benefit, and only caregivers who received the benefit before retirement are allowed to receive it afterwards; benefits stop if the caregiver receives a pension. The caregiver does earn pension rights while receiving the ICA. The program also has a limit on other earnings received by the caregiver. This means that only low-income or temporarily unemployed caregivers will be able to claim the ICA. The average woman who works to support a family cannot. These benefits are so restrictive that it appears that the main purpose of the government is not to support family caregivers as the Swedish do but to save money by getting family members to do the caring at very low compensation rates.

PROPOSALS TO ENCOURAGE FAMILY CARE IN THE UNITED STATES

Several options have been examined by policymakers in the United States to encourage increased sharing of caregiving responsibilities between government and families. These include such programs as paying family members as Medicaid providers of long-term care services, expanding federal tax incentives for informal caregiving, applying the temporary disability insurance model to family caregiving, and making direct payments to caregivers or care recipients.

Families as Medicaid Providers

The program of paying caregivers as Medicaid providers is a popular one, already in use in several states. The federal Medicaid regulations regarding Personal Care prohibit reimbursement of relatives. Therefore, states that do compensate caregivers under Medicaid must do so by utilizing Medicaid Home and Community Based Care waivers. Proponents of paid family caregiving point out that the currently defined compensation regulations under Medicaid for Personal Care Services [CFR 470.170 (f)] could be modified in order to include family caregivers. Other provisions under Medicaid also need to be revised in order to promote family caregiving. For example, an elderly person's SSI and Medicaid benefits are reduced dollar for dollar for any income received from family members. Consequently, there is no incentive for family members to support elderly kin who are receiving such public assistance.

If family members help pay for food, clothing, or shelter for their elderly kin, these payments are also treated as income and if an elderly SSI recipient lives in another person's household and receives free food and shelter from that person, then the recipient is subject to the one-third reduction rule. This rule states that the SSI benefit is reduced by one-third for persons who live in another's household; it can create situations in which an elderly person who lives alone is eligible for Medicaid, whereas others with the same income living in a relative's home are not. Additionally, if elderly SSI recipients do not live with family members, but their families help pay for their food, clothing, and shelter, they are subject to the "presumed value" rule. Under this rule, the total value of the food, shelter, or clothing purchased by family is presumed to be equal to the reduction in SSI benefits made under the one-third reduction rule, unless the recipient can prove that the value is less than this.

Another Medicaid policy is also theorized to encourage separate living arrangements and, therefore, premature institutionalization of elderly SSI recipients. The policy states that the income of spouses is deemed available to the applicant as long as the responsible spouse resides in the same household. This provision can create situations where the individual is ineligible for Medicaid while residing with the caregiver but becomes eligible when living in a separate house or an institution. The 300% rule declares that states may provide Medicaid eligibility to institutionalized persons with incomes up to a certain level as long as that income level does not exceed 300% of the federal SSI benefit level. Thus, elderly persons who are not eligible for Medicaid at home might be if they were to be institutionalized.

As of 1986, 13 states–California, Colorado, Connecticut, Florida, Kansas, Maine, Maryland, Michigan, Minnesota, N. Dakota, Oregon, Virginia, and Wisconsin–provided payments to family caregivers through Medicaid (Burwell, 1986). Brian Burwell lists several reasons that these states support caregivers. Administrators of several state programs, in particular California and Wisconsin, believed that this form of reimbursement provides the recipient a choice of caregiver. Flexibility was also cited as a bonus of these programs. Family caregivers often filled the gaps in professional care. Program administrators also claimed that it was cost effective to pay family members to provide care because they would accept lower wages than a non-relative and the care was believed to be better quality with more personalized attention. Finally, these programs offered support to the caregivers. It was probably not the dollar value of the compensation as much as the positive reinforcement provided that motivated caregivers to continue in their duties, according to Burwell, and "From this perspective, paying family members is a strategy for sustaining the informal caregiving network, not a method for 'purchasing' long-term care services" (Burwell, 1986, p.68).

Tax Incentives

Tax incentives for caregivers comprise another program attractive to policymakers because the tax system is accessible to all persons. These incentives are easy to administer and have a cost-sharing component. There are three basic ways that the government can provide tax incentives, through exemptions, deductions, and credits.

Currently, taxpayers who live with a dependent elderly person may claim that individual as a dependent if the elder has an income of less than $1,000 per year and over half of the support for this elder is provided by the taxpayer. Few persons qualify for this exemption now because of the low income limit placed on the dependent elder. If legislation broadened these provisions and increased the amount of the exemption, it would be of great help to many caregivers. The two primary forms of tax deductions are adjustments to gross income or itemized deductions from taxable income (Burwell, 1986). Tax deductions benefit taxpayers in higher-income brackets, giving them more subsidy per dollar deducted than taxpayers in lower-income brackets (Burwell, 1986).

Less frequently, tax credits are applied directly against a taxpayer's liability. These have the opposite effect of deductions in that they benefit low-income taxpayers more than high-income taxpayers. Currently, a caregiver can claim the Child and Dependent Care Credit provided that the care receiver spends at least eight hours per day in the taxpayer's home and is physically or mentally incapable of caring for his- or herself. All taxpayers in the household must be gainfully employed to receive this credit and expenses are limited to $2,400 per dependent. This method of payment excludes families where one person has the "full-time job" of caregiving.

Expansion of the Temporary Disability Insurance Model

Steven Wisensale (1991) proposes a policy initiative in which the Temporary Disability Insurance (TDI) model would be expanded to include care of family members of all ages by providing an adequate wage replacement to assist family caregivers. To date, only four states (Connecticut, Maine, Washington, and Wisconsin) have enacted legislation that provides leave to care for an elderly parent. But none of these programs offer wage replacement with the family-leave component. Therefore, many caregivers cannot afford the time off. Wisensale proposes that extension of the TDI would consider the family as disabled. He examines the attempt by Massachusetts to implement this type of plan. Resistance to its implementation included the argument that the paid leave would be especially harmful to small business. Even though the bill was defeated, Massachusetts has provided the nation with a new idea for policy initiatives.

Direct Payments

In 1975, U.S. Senate Bill 1161 was introduced and failed as an attempt to provide cash subsidies to families caring for the elderly (Prager, 1978; U.S. Congress, Senate, 1975). Twenty states now provide some type of direct payment to family caregivers with the oldest known direct payment system dating back to 1958 in the state of California (Biegel et al., 1989; Keigher et al., 1988; Linsk, Keigher, & Osterbusch, 1988; Pillemer, MacAdam, & Wolf, 1989). The rest of the programs were implemented in the 1970s and 1980s. As discussed earlier, funding in several states came from the 2176 Medicaid Waiver. David Biegel and his colleagues (1989) found that the payments ranged from an average of $119 per month in Florida to $400 per month in Wisconsin. All of the programs had different requirements for eligibility.

RESEARCH CONCERNING FINANCIAL SUPPORT
FOR FAMILY CAREGIVERS

Although the suggestion of family members' interest in paid family caregiving entered the professional literature in the late 1970s (Sussman, 1977, 1979), there has been little research to determine if financial payments are an effective method for providing support for family caregivers. Some studies report that financial support is not an important factor for most family caregivers of the elderly (Arling & McAuley, 1983; Cantor, 1983; Horowitz & Shindelman, 1983). Amy Horowitz and Lois Shindelman (1983) reported extremely negative reactions from a significant number of family caregivers who refused to even consider financial support. The researchers asked caregivers to rank their preferences for various service and economic support programs; they then compared their findings to those of Marvin B. Sussman's 1977 and 1979 studies. Sussman indicated that medical care was the preferred service support while the monthly check was the preferred financial program. When all programs were considered together, the majority of Sussman's respondents chose the monthly check as the most desirable. But, Horowitz and Shindelman pointed out that Sussman's sample consisted primarily of individuals who were not actually caregivers but were responding to hypothetical questions only. Horowitz and Shindelman also found that in the general category of economic incentives, including tax incentives, food stamps, monthly checks and home improvement loans, the monthly check was by far the preferred form of support. This study differed somewhat from Sussman's findings in that the group in the Horowitz and Shindelman study was split as to what service they preferred. Half of the sample preferred medical care and the other half chose homemaking services. The service category also included programs such as community planning services, respite care, and a social center for the elder. The respite care service was seen as the least critical for the caregivers.

The remarkable difference occurred when the Horowitz and Shindelman sample was asked to choose just one program. Over 80% chose a service rather than a financial support. These results are extremely important in light of the fact that most of the programs currently in use or proposed for implementation by the government include some type of financial incentive. Research shows that the financial strains seem to be of less consequence to the caregivers than the physical and emotional strains they experience. Just because the financial concerns are not the primary ones mentioned by caregivers does not mean that they are not burdensome. These results point to the necessity for a combination of service and financial supports for caregivers.

CONCLUSION

This article has presented an overview of the current debate on policies to support family caregiving. In Western Europe, particularly Sweden and the United Kingdom, initiatives are now in place. Supports include a care leave policy implemented at the federal level, paying caregiver salaries to family members when caregiving is a full-time job, providing job training to salaried caregivers when their personal caregiving experience ends, community-based programs for caregivers, and allowances to be used for care of an elderly or disabled person. In the United States as of 1986, 13 states paid caregivers as Medicaid providers. Policymakers have considered tax incentives and, in 1975, U.S. Senate Bill 1161 was introduced and failed as an attempt to provide cash subsidies to families caring for the elderly. Wisensale (1991) proposes expanding the Temporary Disability Model to include care of family members of all ages by providing adequate wage replacement to assist family caregivers. As of 1989, 34 states provided some type of economic support for caregivers (Biegel & Blum, 1990).

The literature focuses on these macro-level solutions to caregiving problems while neglecting the creative solutions that families can devise at the micro-level. Such topics are just beginning to be addressed in the literature. The family's internal financial arrangements, such as "inheritance contracting" (Hanks & Sussman, 1991) or sharing of care and financial outlay for parents by a sibling group (Cicirelli, 1991) are examples of solutions. As suggested by Eugene Litwak (1985), there are some services that may be better performed by family members and some that are more efficiently handled by formal organizations. Research needs to be done to determine what types of programs are most acceptable and beneficial to caregivers as well as cost effective for federal, state, and local governments.

There is a growing need for care of the elderly and if society expects the family to care for its elders, then public and private support must be available. Supporting caregivers in their difficult task can prevent premature or unnecessary institutionalization of the elderly and cut the rising costs of medical care to the institutionalized elderly.

REFERENCES

Arling, G., & McAuley, W.J. (1983). The feasibility of public payments for family caregiving. *The Gerontologist, 23* (3), 300-306.

Barberis, M. (1981). America's elderly: Policy implications. *Population Bulletin, 35* (4), Policy Supplement. Washington, DC: Population Reference Bureau.

Biegel, D.E., Schultz, R., Shore, B.K., & Morycz, R. (1989). Economic supports for family caregivers of the elderly: Public sector policies. In M. Z. Goldstein, (Ed.), *Family involvement in treatment of the frail elderly* (159-201). Washington, DC: American Psychiatric Press.

Biegel, D. E., & Blum, A. (Eds.) (1990). *Aging and caregiving: Theory, research, and policy.* Newbury Park, CA: Sage.

Brody, E. (1981). Women in the middle and family help to older people. *The Gerontologist, 21* (5), 471-480.

Brody, E. (1985). Parent care as a normative family stress. *The Gerontologist, 25* (1), 19-29.

Burwell, B.O. (1986). *Shared obligations: Public policy influences on family care for the elderly.* Working Paper (No. 500-83-0056). Washington, DC: Department of Health and Human Services, Health Care Financing Administration, Office of Research and Demonstrations, SysteMetrics/McGraw-Hill, Inc.

Cantor, M.H. (1983). Strain among caregivers: A study of experience in the United States. *The Gerontologist, 23* (6), 597-604.

Cicirelli, V.G. (1991). Sibling relationships in adulthood. In S.K. Pfiefer & M.B. Sussman (Eds.), *Families: Intergenerational and generational connections.* Binghamton, NY: The Haworth Press, Inc.

Coberly, S. (1991). *An employer's guide to eldercare.* Washington, DC: Washington Business Group on Health, Institute on Aging, Work, & Health.

Deimling, G.T., & Bass, D.M. (1986). Symptoms of mental impairment among elderly adults and their effects on family caregivers. *Journal of Gerontology, 41* (6), 778-784.

England, S., Linsk, N.L., Simon-Rusinowitz, L., & Keigher, S.M. (1989). Paid family caregiving and the market view of home care: Agency perspectives. *Journal of Health and Social Policy, 1* (2), 31-53.

England, S.E., Linsk, N.L., Simon-Rusinowitz, L.S., & Keigher, S.M. (1990). Paying kin for care: Agency barriers to formalizing informal care. *Journal of Aging & Social Policy, 2* (2), 63-86.

Fengler, A.P., & Goodrich, N. (1979). Wives of elderly disabled men: The hidden patients. *The Gerontologist, 19* (2), 175-183.

George, L.K., & Gwyther, L.P. (1986). Caregiver well-being: A multi-dimensional examination of family caregivers of demented adults. *The Gerontologist, 26* (3), 253-259.

Gilhooly, M.L.M. (1984). The impact of caregiving on caregivers: Factors associated with the psychological well-being of people supporting a demented relative in the community. *British Journal of Medical Psychology, 57,* 35-44.

Grana, J.M. (1983). Disability allowances for long-term care in Western Europe and the United States. *International Social Security Review, 36* (2), 207-221.

Haley, W.E., Levine, E.G., Brown, S.L., & Bartolucci, A.A. (1987). Stress, appraisal, coping, and social supports as predictors of adaptational outcome among dementia caregivers. *Psychology and Aging, 2* (4), 323-330.

Haley, W.E., Levine, E.G., Brown, S.L., Berry, J.W., & Hughes, G.H. (1987). Psychological, social and health consequences of caring for a relative with senile dementia. *Journal of the American Geriatrics Society, 35,* 405-411.

Hanks, R.S., & Sussman, M.B. (1991, November). Inheritance contracting: Implications for theory and policy. Paper presented at the Pre-Conference Workshop on Theory Construction and Research Methodology, Annual Conference of the National Council on Family Relations, Denver, CO.

Hokenstad, M.C., & Johansson, L. (1990a). Caregiving for the elderly in Sweden. In D. E. Biegel and A. Blum, (Eds.), *Aging and caregiving: Theory, research and policy,* Beverly Hills: Sage.

Hokenstad, M.C. & Johansson, L. (1990b). Swedish policy initiatives to support family caregiving for the elderly. *Ageing International, 17* (1), 33-35.

Hooyman, N.R., & Lustbader, W. (1986). *Taking care: Supporting older people and their families.* New York: Free Press.

Horowitz, A., & Shindelman, L.W. (1983). Social and economic incentives for family caregivers. *Health Care Financing Review, 5* (2), 25-33.

Jones, D.A., & Vetter, N.J. (1984). A survey of those who care for the elderly at home: Their problems and their needs. *Social Science and Medicine, 19* (5), 511-514.

Keigher, S. M. (1991). Wages or welfare? Compensating caregiving in two conservative social welfare states. *Journal of Aging & Social Policy, 3* (3), 83-104.

Keigher, S.M., Simon-Rusinowitz, L.S., Linsk, N.L., & Osterbusch, S.E. (1988). Payments to informal versus formal home care providers: Policy divergence affecting the elderly and their families in Michigan and Illinois. *Journal of Applied Gerontology, 7* (4), 456-473.

Kosberg, J.I. (1988). Preventing elder abuse: Identification of high risk factors prior to placement decisions. *The Gerontologist, 28* (1), 43-57.

Krause, A., Spasoff, R., Beattie, E., Holden, E., Lawson, J., Rodenberg, M., &

Woodcock, G. (1976). Elderly applicants to long-term care institutions. *Journal of the American Geriatrics Society, 24*, 117-125.

Linsk, N.L., Keigher, S.M., & Osterbusch, S.E. (1988). States' policies regarding paid family caregiving. *The Gerontologist, 28* (2), 204-212.

Litwak, E. (1985). *Helping the elderly: The complementary roles of informal networks and formal systems.* New York: Guilford Press.

Manton, K.G. (1986). Past and future life expectancy increases at later ages: Their implications for the linkage of chronic morbidity, disability, and mortality. *Journals of Gerontology, 41* (5), 672-681.

Morris, R., & Bass, S.A. (Eds.) (1988). *Retirement reconsidered: Economic and social roles for older people.* New York: Springer Publishing Company.

Morycz, R.K. (1985). Caregiving strain and the desire to institutionalize family members with Alzheimer's disease. *Research on Aging, 7* (3), 329-361.

Neal, M.B., Chapman, N.J., Ingersoll-Dayton, B., Emlen, A.C., & Boise, L. (1990). Absenteeism and stress among employed caregivers of the elderly, disabled adults, and children. In D. Bigel and A. Blum (Eds.), *Aging & Caregiving: Theory, research, and policy.* Newbury Park, CA: Sage.

Pearlman, D.N., & Crown, W.H. (1992). Alternative sources of social support and their impact on institutional risk. *The Gerontologist, 32* (4), 527-535.

Pifer, A., & Bronte, L. (1986). *Our aging society.* New York: W.W. Norton.

Pillemer, K., MacAdam, M., & Wolf, R.S. (1989). Services to families with dependent elders. *Journal of Aging & Social Policy, 1* (3/4), 67-88.

Prager, E. (1978). Subsidized family care of the aged: U.S. Senate Bill 1161. *Policy Analysis, 4*, 477-490.

Rabins, P.V., Mace, N.L., & Lucas, M.J. (1982). The impact of dementia on the family. *Journal of the American Medical Association, 248* (3), 333-335.

Robinson, B., & Thurnher, M. (1979). Taking care of aged parents: A family cycle transition. *The Gerontologist, 19*, 586-593.

Rosenwaike, I. (1985). *The extreme aged in America.* Westport, CT: Greenwood Press.

Ross, H., & Kedward, H. (1977). Psychogeriatric hospital admission from the community and institutions. *Journals of Gerontology, 32*, 420-427.

Stone, R. (1987). Exploding the myths: Caregiving in America (One Hundredth Congress, First Session. Select Committee on Aging, U.S. House of Representatives Comm. Pub. No. 99-611). Washington, DC: U.S. Government Printing Office.

Sheehan, N.W., & Nuttall, P. (1988). Conflict, emotion, and personal strain among family caregivers. *Family Relations, 37*, 92-98.

Simon-Rusinowitz, L. (1987). Government participation in long-term care of the elderly: Analysis of a policy to pay family caregivers. Unpublished doctoral dissertation. University of Illinois at Chicago.

Social Security Administration. (1989). *Social Security Bulletin, Annual Statistical Supplement, 1989.* Washington, DC: U.S. Government Printing Office.

Stone, R. (1987). Exploding the myths: Caregiving in America. U.S. House Select Committee on Aging, U.S. House of Representatives. (100th Congress, First

Session. Comm. Pub. No. 99-611). Washington, DC: U.S. Government Printing Office.

Sussman, M.B. (1977). *Incentives and family environment for the elderly.* Final Report to Administration on Aging. Grant No. 90-A-316. February, 1977. Washington, DC: Administration on Aging.

Sussman, M.B. (1979). *Social and economic supports and family environments for the elderly.* Final Report to Administration on Aging. Grant No. 90-A-316(03) January, 1979. Washington, DC: Administration on Aging.

Tobin, S., & Kulys, R. (1981). The family in the institutionalization of the elderly. *Journal of Social Issues, 37,* 145-157.

U.S.A. Today. (1992, April 9). How families will cope with an aging population, page 11A.

U.S. Bureau of the Census. (1990). *Statistical Abstract of the United States, 1990* (110th ed.). Washington, DC: U.S. Government Printing Office.

U.S. House Select Committee on Aging, U.S. House of Representatives. (100th Congress, First Session. Comm. Pub. No. 99-611). Washington, DC: U.S. Government Printing Office. U.S. Senate (1975). *Congressional Record,* 94th Congress, 1st session, March 12, 1975, 121(3).

Wade, A. (1984). *Social Security Area Population Projections, 1984.* Social Security Administration. Actuarial Study No. 92.

Wagner, D.L., Creedon, M.A., Sasala, J.M., & Neal, M.B. (1989). *Employees and eldercare: Designing effective responses for the workplace.* Prepared for Workplace Responses to Eldercare Teleconference, September 22, 1989. Presented by University of Bridgeport National Council on the Aging.

Wisensale, S.K. (1991). An intergenerational policy proposal for the 1990s: Applying the temporary disability insurance model to family caregiving. *Journal of Aging & Social Policy, 3* (1/2), 163-183.

Zarit, S.H., Reever, K.E., & Bach-Peterson, J. (1980). Relatives of the impaired elderly: Correlates of feelings of burden. *The Gerontologist, 20* (6), 260-266.

Caregiving and Long-Term Health Care in the People's Republic of China

Philip Olson, PhD

University of Missouri-Kansas City

SUMMARY. The growing proportion of frail elderly in the People's Republic of China has necessitated policy of the state toward their long-term care. In this decade, there has been an increase in the amount of data available on the care and needs of Chinese frail elders. This article synthesizes these data and traces the patterns of care of frail elders. It distinguishes between urban and rural patterns, and identifies the increasing role of the family and community in the caregiving of elders. State policy, evident from the data, suggests that the state's role in direct care of elders is minor but that it continues to influence and support eldercare as part of its policy of promoting the one-child per couple policy. This process can be seen in support programs for the childless elder, who symbolizes the expected condition of a large number of future elders under the one-child policy. The article identifies four factors that are influencing the changing patterns of long-term care of elders in China: (1) economic reform programs; (2) the political agenda of the Chinese Communist Party; (3) differences in urban and rural economic conditions; and (4) policy directed at long-term investment in health care technology.

Philip Olson is Professor of Sociology and Director of Urban Affairs at the University of Missouri-Kansas City; he is also Adjunct Professor of Sociology at Shanghai University, People's Republic of China (PRC). Dr. Olson is engaged in a long-term study of the elderly in the PRC and has made four research trips there since 1981. His research has been published in aging journals and as chapters in special volumes devoted to aging in non-American cultures.

[Haworth co-indexing entry note]: "Caregiving and Long-Term Health Care in the People's Republic of China," Olson, Philip. Co-published simultaneously in the *Journal of Aging & Social Policy,* (The Haworth Press, Inc.) Vol. 5, No. 1/2, 1993, pp. 91-110; and: *International Perspectives on State and Family Support for the Elderly* (ed: Scott A. Bass and Robert Morris) The Haworth Press, Inc., 1993, pp. 91-110. Multiple copies of this article/chapter may be purchased from The Haworth Document Delivery Center [1-800-3-HAWORTH; 9:00 a.m. - 5:00 p.m. (EST)].

91

China is commonly viewed as a society that reveres its elderly. Filial piety reportedly has existed for centuries, undergirded by the teachings of Confucianism. China is often portrayed as the paramount example of obedience to the elder and of political and social rule by the old. However, the ideals and public images of a society are often quite different from the realities of its daily life. The actual treatment and regard for elders can be influenced by factors other than the traditional values of that society.

In China, elders are not always given the respect and reverence that tradition dictates. Evidence exists of elder abuse, inadequate housing conditions for some childless elders, inadequate retirement programs for some urban elders, and virtually no retirement plan for rural elders (Chen, 1970; Macciocchi, 1972; Olson, 1987). Examination of various historical periods reveals that elders were sometimes discriminated against by political regimes, or by the day-to-day activities of other age groups. In fact, the most well-known period in modern China's history, the Cultural Revolution (1966-1975), was a period in which all those, including the elderly, who represented the traditional values of the past were persecuted.

This article is an effort to examine the relationship of social, economic, and political factors to the care and treatment of frail elders in China during the period following the death of Mao Zedong. This analysis explores factors other than traditional values that affect policies toward and treatment of the frail elderly. Specifically, the effects of the political economy on health care of the frail elderly are examined. The frail elderly are the most vulnerable segment of elderly in the society; they are those needing health care and assistance with daily living because of physical and mental disabilities. Their treatment by the society reflects most clearly the effects of government policy in a state-controlled economy such as China (Wolf, 1986). In the 15 years since Mao's death, major reforms occurring in the Communist Party and in the political economy of China have shaped policies and programs aimed at the care of elders.

MODERNIZATION POLICIES IN POST-MAO CHINA

The death of Mao Zedong in 1976 brought an end to efforts to develop a completely state-controlled economy. The new era was marked by full-scale modernization. In January 1975, Premier Zhou En-lai announced the Four Modernizations Program and set as a target date for its achievement the year 2000. The program centered on the development of agriculture, the military, industry, and science and technology. The adoption of the program in 1978 promoted China's development through technological growth rather than through class struggle, as the "cultural revolution" had attempted.

Three major reform efforts during the modernization efforts of the 1980s and 1990s have affected long-term care policies and other conditions of the elderly population.

Population Reform. Among the first policies reformulated following Mao's death was population reform; the new policy was aimed at further reduction in the growth of population as a necessary step in economic reform (Saith, 1981). Unless population growth could be stopped, economic development could never be realized because the growing population would erode gains in economic growth. Although population control began as early as 1962, its impact was not substantial until the "one-child" per couple policy became fully operational in the early 1980s (Kallgren, 1985; Wolf, 1986). In the decade since its inception, it has shown dramatic signs of success, largely in urban areas and in those rural counties closely linked to urban centers along the eastern coast of China (Bianco, 1981; Chen, 1985; Poston & Gu, 1984).

Economic Reform. The political successor to Mao, Deng Xiaoping, "encouraged unity through increased economic interdependence, through reliance on effective, planned allocation of material goods and capital, and through a regularized promotion and personnel management system" (Oksenberg, 1982, p. 170). The decade of the 1980s witnessed a remarkable reform of the entire economy, including the abolition of the farm commune, the opening of "free markets" for many goods and services, the institutionalization of a work-incentive policy, greater decentralization of enterprise management, implementation of a mixed controlled and market economy, and greater reliance on Western technology, capital, and markets. Most of the economic indicators available suggest that the economic reform efforts have resulted in growth in nearly all parts of the system, large-scale improvements in the standard of living, inflation, and greater "Westernization" of the lifestyles of the Chinese peoples, especially those living in urban areas. It has been suggested, however, that there continue to be inequities between rural and urban elders, and the principal reason for those inequities is the unwillingness of the central government leaders to break from the policy "that defines most social welfare goods as rewards to job statuses and thereby allocates the best quality services to the most highly ranked employees," who live in cities (Davis 1989, p. 581).

Party Reform. Begun in the early 1980s, the major political reforms included abolishing life tenure for cadres, encouraging retirement of veteran cadres, and promoting younger cadres to leading posts (An, 1982). In a speech delivered in 1981 on the occasion of the 60th anniversary of the founding of the Chinese Communist Party, Party Chairman Hu Yaobang said, "It is now a pressing strategic task facing the whole party to build up a large contingent of revolutionary, well-educated, professionally competent and younger cadres . . . and they [old, veteran cadres] should free themselves from the onerous pressure of day-to-day work. . . . " (Liu 1986, p. 355). A major thrust of party reform has been to streamline the bulging bureaucracy, often cited as a cause of the sluggishness of the reform, the major impediment to efficiency, and a drain on the economy. This policy was launched in 1982 when the Party Central Committee passed a resolution establishing a veteran cadre retirement system (Zhao, 1987). In the words of Deng, the goals are "to make the ranks of cadres more revolutionary, younger in average age, better educated, and more professionally competent" (Deng, 1983). In 1983, over 800,000 veteran cadres retired, signaling that the new retirement policy was under way (Ding, 1984).

THE STATE AND THE FRAIL ELDERLY

The three major reforms outlined above, though aimed at economic and political change, have significant consequences for China's elderly population, especially its frail elderly. China is currently faced with a growing proportion of frail elders while at the same time struggling to meet the needs of a very large younger population and directing resources into modernization efforts. The growth in the frail elderly population creates a dilemma for the state. Frail elders require resources for their care, both human and material; a political economy that is struggling to modernize by putting most of its resources into capital growth must weigh how to allocate resources to its nonproductive members. How can it keep true to its tradition of reverence for its elders while moving forward with its modernization efforts, especially during times when resources remain scarce?

Frail Elderly in China

The modernization of China contributes to the increase in the proportion and number of older persons in that society. Modernization theory attributes this growth in the elderly population to improved hygiene, health care, diets, and other socio-medical changes (Cowgill, 1986). In 1985, China's over-65-year-old population constituted 5% of the total population. Within 30 years, by 2015, it will double to 10% (Banister, 1988, p. 75). The very old, those over 80, constituted 11% of the over-65 population in 1985 and by 2015 will grow to 19% (Banister, 1988, p. 75), nearly one fifth of all elders. It is those elders over age 80 who are most likely to need health care and other assistance as their frailty increases.

An emphasis on the frail elderly in the following discussion is important because frail elders highlight the issue of competing interests on the systems of support. The dilemma presented by this constituency involves defining, through social policy, how resources should be allocated among the nonproductive sectors of the domestic publics. It raises the question: How does the political system allocate resources among the needs of the youth, the needs for stability of the family, the need for continued economic growth, the development of the vast peasant society, and the need to care for elders? Frail elders, who can offer little or no return on the investment in their long-term care, are in an especially unusual and important position in a society that is struggling with its economic development.

The Political Economy Perspective

In attempting to understand the issues surrounding social and economic change and their influence on a population such as frail elders, it has been argued that sociologists have long overlooked the state as a variable (Skocpol, 1985). However, this appears to be changing: others factor in the role of the state in pointing out that welfare for the elder population, in the form of retirement pensions, is found primarily in capitalistic societies (Myles, 1984). Carroll Estes and colleagues (1984) focus on the political economy, and identify it as the overriding factor in determining how eldercare is addressed.

"Political economy" refers to the economic system that is supported and promoted by the political system that has garnered the power to operate the government and thus regulate or control the economy. The question of how economic growth gets transformed into expenditures is a central issue of the political economy perspective (Estes et al., 1984). This perspective highlights the fact that in the United States, health care is a part of the market economy, and the management of illness is a business. Furthermore, eldercare is an integral part of that market economy. Since the ethos of the U.S. political economy is profit and growth, the system is benefitted when the aging population is defined in terms of its illness rather than in terms of its wellness.

In China, however, the health care system is not a central part of the economy, and illness is not defined as an element of economic growth. While the health care system in China is a necessary system and is being modernized along with other sectors, health care technology and training are costly investments. There is no advantage for there to be a large "sick" population in China. Developing societies, like China, first address problems of communicable diseases. Only when these diseases have been controlled does attention turn to dealing with chronic diseases, which are not only costly to the society but focus largely on the older population. In China, this issue is now before the government. "Success in the control of communicable disease has transferred the burden of China's health problems to the older age groups. . . . Prevention is relatively difficult for most chronic diseases, and development of effective, yet low-cost, strategies for dealing with these disorders is a priority. The major pitfall is the temptation to emulate high-cost curative approaches that have proved relatively inefficacious and that, even in high-income countries, have resulted in a massive drain on national economic resources" (Jamison, Evans, & King 1984, p. xvii). How China deals with its frail elder population is then a reflection of the political decisions on how that "problem" is defined.

Others suggest that policies of development are in part influenced by how the aged population is defined relative to economic development (Treas & Logue, 1986). They identify four perspectives societies use to define their aged: (1) as a low priority; (2) as an impediment; (3) as a resource; or (4) as victims of the development process. Most developing societies regard their older population from more than one perspective: in China the old are publicly hailed as resources who can play an important role in the development of the society (China News Analysis, 1984; Ikels, 1990b). Yet an examination of current programs for elders suggests they are a low priority in the allocation of public resources.

Role of the State and the Family in Eldercare

Consistent with its ideology of minimizing illness and maximizing self-sufficiency, the government and the Communist Party promote local initiatives that foster a minimum role for the state and a maximum role for the family and community in eldercare, especially for the very old, the frail, and the dependent (Henderson, 1990; Ikels, 1990a). The development of modernization in China under Communism, together with the political intervention of the Chinese Communist Party, have reinforced the role of the family and have clarified the balance of responsibility between the state and the family for eldercare, especially during the 1980s (Whyte & Parish, 1984; Wolf, 1986).

In traditional China, both rural and urban, the extended family was the primary unit that provided for elders. In the current period, while the family remains a central element in care of elders, other factors influence the role of the family. A major factor is the rural-urban distinction. In 1982, 80% of China's population was rural. Although, according to the 1990 Chinese census, the rural population dropped to 73.8%, China remains predominantly rural and agricultural. In addition to a predominantly rural population, China's economy is bifurcated. This dual economy has endured through the 30 years of Communism, with the urban sector becoming semi-modernized and receiving about 70% of the state investment, while the rural sector continues to depend on local surpluses. More comprehensive social and health care services accrue to urban elders because of subsidization from the state; in rural areas social and health services are primarily the result of "regeneration through one's own efforts" (*zi li geng sheng*) (Davis-Friedmann, 1984, p. 207). Such a dual economy has led to very different policies and programming for rural and urban frail elders, reflecting the very different roles of the family and the state in long-term care in each setting.

In rural areas, parents expect to guarantee their care in old age through a married son who will provide for them in the absence of a pension system and other social services. Family reciprocity is the basic system that ensures eldercare in rural areas. Living with a married son offers both economic and social security for the elder, and in exchange, the elder contributes to the household economy through childcare, gardening, and household work.

In urban areas, where 75% of all adults are state employees, parents look to the state to provide for them through a retirement pension and social services, and children are seen as dependents rather than as supports. Because of seniority, older workers receive more pay than younger workers, and the additional household income earned by elders is often used to subsidize expenses of children through household purchases, gifts for grandchildren, vacations, and medical expenses (Davis-Friedmann, 1985b; Sankar, 1989). However, despite the fact that the state in urban areas plays a major role in providing economic support for the aged, the family still provides the majority of eldercare. Studies done in two of the largest cities in China reported that when elders became ill, in Tianjin 96% of them were cared for directly by family members, and in Beijing 87% received care from family members (Yuan, 1987).

Health Care of the Frail Elders

Of particular importance is how a society addresses the health and long-term care needs of those chronically ill and frail elders unable to care for themselves. Long-term care as defined here includes the continuum of activities directed toward the physical, medical, and social care of persons unable to provide for themselves. It includes institutional care as well as in-home family care, and is provided by both skilled personnel as well as family members, friends, or neighbors.

Though the principal support for elders, including frail elders, is the family unit, other health care supports supplement the family. These supports in China are, however, much less extensive than one would expect given its long tradition of respect toward elders. As early as 1983, observers of social welfare policies in China noted that the overall intention of China was, "to avoid the creation of large welfare agencies which have drained the capacity of richer governments" (China News Analysis, 1984, p. 8). The family and local communal organizations are expected to provide much of the long-term care for frail elders, thus preventing costly institutionalization. This policy is evident in both rural and urban areas, although the higher standard of living and the generally better medical care in urban areas conceals the extent to which urban areas rely on these informal support systems. The major exception to this policy in both rural and urban areas are the childless elderly, who receive special benefits.

In rural China, health care for both acute and chronically ill frail elders is available through primary health care stations, rural hospitals, "barefoot doctors," nurse aides, and some "nursemaids" (*bao mu*) (Davis-Friedmann, 1984; Jamison, Evans, & King, 1984; Liang & Gu, 1989).

Primary health care stations are clinics operated in small quarters of existing public buildings or sometimes in separate structures. These stations are in small villages, and there are also larger clinics in the township (*xiang*). The village stations contain basic medical-examination features, but provide little privacy to the patient. Medical treatment includes traditional medicine (herbal medicine) and acupuncture. Treatment depends on the diagnosis and preference of the attending doctor and the patient. Minor illnesses and injuries are treated and immunizations administered (Hu, 1984). A typical staff includes two or three doctors and one or more nurses. The stations keep regular hours, but are also available on an emergency basis. There is great variance in the size and equipment of these stations.

In wealthier areas, particularly in agricultural areas along the eastern coastal region, facilities are substantial and include equipment such as X-ray machines. In the poorer counties, there may be little more than a sparsely furnished room with no equipment. In the mid-1980s over half of these rural stations were privately operated by village doctors and only four percent supported by the state (Ministry of Public Health, 1986). In 1986 among the 7.38 million villages in China, there were approximately 6.48 million primary health stations (Liang & Gu, 1989, p. 277).

The village doctor, sometimes referred to as a "barefoot doctor," is typically a peasant with a primary school education, receiving three to six months of medical training and qualified to treat minor diseases and injuries. He also oversees local public health workers. The name derives from the fact that many of these people are peasants who dress and live much like the rural peasants. In 1986, there were estimated to be 12.8 million village doctors (Liang & Gu, 1989, p. 277). Herbal medicine and traditional measures like acupuncture are widespread and low-cost measures are administered by them as well as by the primary health care stations. However, the decollectivization of agriculture has been accompanied by a decline in the number of village health clinics and these practitioners–now called "countryside doctors." Between 1975 (the year with the highest number of barefoot doctors) and 1986, their numbers declined 18% and the total number of village health personnel declined by more than 50% (Henderson, 1990, p. 271).

Nursemaids (*bao mu*) are semiskilled workers in health care who are hired by families to take care of a bedridden person either in the hospital or at home. To keep hospital costs low, nursing staffing is limited, and it is expected that family members will be present at the bedside of the sick relative most of the time. To relieve the family burden, the family may hire nursemaids to perform this task; they are also hired for in-home care of frail elders who are bed-bound.

Some rural areas have adopted the *bao hu zu* (voluntary nursing service), in which supervised in-home care is done by neighbor volunteers who are sometimes paid minimally for their services. In many small villages, a local committee signs a "guaranteed community service agreement with nearby neighbors, schools, or other service units to provide certain services such as delivery of groceries, medicines, or coal, and regular monitoring of the health status of frail childless elders" (Zhu, 1990, pp. 2-3).

Reflecting the dual economy, health services in rural areas are not as advanced as in urban areas. In 1986, the number of hospital beds per 1,000 persons in rural areas was 1.54, compared to 4.48 in urban areas–nearly three times as many (Henderson, 1990, p. 270). Hospitals are generally a unit of the county, and care is primarily for short-term and acute illnesses. Patients who cannot be adequately treated at the primary health care stations in the *xiang* (township) are sent to the county hospital.

The services described here are designed primarily to supplement family care for the frail and chronically ill elder. This situation is changing under the economic reforms brought about in the early 1980s. The change, however, is toward *reduced* health services in rural areas, increased costs, and fragmented programs of health insurance from one rural area to another (Henderson, 1990). Retrenchment places more responsibility on the family unit.

The major exception to these trends in health care for frail elders in rural areas is the policy toward the childless elderly. The policy has two parts: the *wu bao hu*, five guarantee households (described earlier), and *jing lao yuan*, homes for the aged (Zhang, 1986). During the last 10 years, thousands of homes for the aged have been built. The government reported an increase from 7,825 homes in 1978 to 33,295 in 1986 (*Shehui Baozhang Bao,* April 10, 1987) and an increase to 36,665 in 1988 (*Social Statistics of China, 1990*). These homes serve as a symbol to rural families that when there is no family member to care for them in old age, the community will provide care. As others have noted, these homes also function to reinforce the one-child policy by reassuring young families who fear that having only one child will increase their risk of having no one to provide for them in their old age (Davis-Friedmann, 1985a; Ikels, 1990a; Olson, 1987; Zhang, 1986).

Criteria for admission to a home are that the person (1) has no living children near enough to provide care; (2) is not bedridden or requiring constant medical care; (3) is willing to enter the home; and (4) qualifies for local welfare assistance (*wu bao*). Typically, a local committee monitors the status of older childless persons and determines when "the time has come" for them to be admitted to the local *jing lao yuan*. A committee member who knows the person visits with them and suggests the idea; typically, it takes a few visits to get them to "come around" to seeing that it is best to be in the home. Once in the home, should long-term hospitalization or medical care be needed, the person is sent to a county hospital.

The China National Committee on Aging, a governmental unit, has been engaged in a campaign to promote the establishment of *jing lao yuan* in every rural township throughout China (Olson, 1988, pp. 253-254). Yet, even though it is national government policy to develop supports for childless elders, the financing of these measures is left largely to the local governmental unit. Each township is expected to design, build, administer, and maintain at least one *jing lao yuan*.

In urban areas, fragmentary data from a number of small-scale surveys done in different cities in China give some hint of the magnitude of long-term care issues for the urban aged. A study done in Shanghai in 1985 indicates that the proportion of those needing long-term care increases with age (Yu, Liu, Levy, & Zhang, 1989). For those aged 75 and over, 10.5% can engage in activities only with help compared to less than 1% (0.7%) of those aged 55 to 64.

Some researchers believe that perceived health status is yet another measure of the degree to which a population may be described as needing long-term care. From the Shanghai study, the proportion of those who perceived themselves to be in poor health was nearly one fifth of the total population aged 75 and over. A 1987 study of the elderly in Guangzhou shows that of those with self-reported impairments, half or more of those over age 85 indicated moderate or major impairments in vision, mobility, and mental functioning (Ikels, 1990a).

There are special provisions of welfare and health assistance from the state to certain groups of urban elders needing long-term care, including the childless, nonstate employees, and a small number of others. However, the majority of assistance to urban elders comes through direct assistance from one's work unit (*dan wei*), or one's community unit, the Street Station (*jia dao*). All state employees, about 75% of all urban workers, are covered by health insurance, which carries over into retirement. It covers most medical care, but doesn't provide for long-term care. In 1986, the program added a co-payment, requiring 5% to 10% payment for medication and hospitalization. In addition, several expensive procedures were no longer covered (Ikels, 1990a, p. 280). This policy has shifted slightly the burden of health care away from the state to the individual. Disabilities that force workers to retire prior to retirement age are compensated for both by a retirement pension and a stipend to employ a *bao mu.* The amount of money depends on the length of employment by the disabled worker, but it is a lifetime guarantee (Davis-Friedmann, 1985b, p. 306). Except for the addition of a co-payment, recent analyses indicate that there have been only minor changes in medical care benefits for retired workers during the 1980s (Liu, 1990, p. 20).

Economic reforms during the 1980s that have led to a reduction of health care services for rural elders have resulted in increases in some services to urban elders. There has been growth in hospital construction, in high-tech equipment such as CT scanners, and in the number of health care personnel during the late 1980s (Henderson, 1990, pp. 269-271).

Long-term care in urban areas for the childless has basically two components: (1) social welfare institutes (operated by the Bureau of Civil Affairs), which are the urban counterpart to the rural *jing lao yuan* and where well elderly as well as frail, bedridden, and elders needing total care live permanently; and (2) community-based in-home care (*bao hu zhu*) (Liang & Gu, 1989; Sankar, 1989; Zhu, 1990).

Social welfare institutes vary in size, function, and financing, depending on the city. Shanghai (the largest city in China with a population of more than 16 million people) has the most well-developed facilities in urban China. The overall rate of growth of these facilities throughout China has not been significant; in 1978 there were 577 homes and by 1985 the number had risen to 752. However, the expenditure per capita did rise significantly from 553 yuan (approximately $166 U.S.) in 1978 to 1782 yuan (approximately $535 U.S.) by 1985 (Liu, 1989b, p. 113), but much of this increase may be accounted for by inflation.

Urban welfare institutes provide the same kind of services as rural *jing lao yuan,* though their physical plants are very different.

The urban facilities are often multistoried, whereas the rural homes are single-storied and have a garden-like environment.

Community-based in-home care in urban areas is developing rapidly. Under this program, the Street Station (*jia dao*) has responsibility for administering the funds it receives from the municipal government by passing them on to the Resident's Committees that serve local neighborhoods. These local Resident's Committees identify childless elders and others needing in-home care, and train and supervise a person who is assigned to regularly visit, prepare meals, run errands, notify the doctor, and in other ways attend to the needs of the homebound elder. This system, called *bao hu zu*, has been operating only since the early 1980s (Liang & Gu, 1989, p. 274; Olson, 1987, pp. 291-292;) but grew dramatically during the late 1980s. According to one set of data, for all of China there were 36,000 persons in 1986 looking after 66,000 persons; by 1988 these had grown to 54,000 caring for 88,000 older persons (Zhu, 1990, p. 1). The kinds of services vary from short-term volunteer in-home care to exchanges between household units in which the elder provides household services to a younger working family in return for care during his or her times of illness (Liang & Gu, 1989, p. 274; Zhu, 1990, p. 2).

In addition to the welfare institutes and the *bao hu zu*, frail elders are cared for through a variety of other means. There are organized efforts of students, military personnel, factory employees, and local government employees to provide such assistance as home repair, carrying of heavy supplies, and home decorating (Liang & Gu, 1989, p. 274; Olson, 1987, pp. 287-288). Another approach, one that is relatively new, is the "home-based sick bed" (Henderson, 1990, p. 290). A medical care organization, such as a hospital, designates the sick bed. The designation of sick bed means that services, under the management of a doctor, are provided to the elder in his or her own home. An elder seeking medical care at a neighborhood clinic or hospital will be designated eligible for a home sick bed, after having been examined, if he or she is not sick enough for in-hospital care, but too sick to be sent home with only medicine. The practice is designed primarily for persons with chronic illnesses, those who are convalescing or those who need rehabilitation. Services offered in the sick-bed system include drug therapy, physical therapy, nutrition, exams, mental health counseling, and traditional Chinese treatments (Liang & Gu, 1989, p. 277). The number of sick beds in operation rose from 490,000 in 1984 to 831,000 in 1986 (Liang & Gu, 1989, p. 277). Of major significance is the cost savings; savings of 37% to 57% over the use of hospital beds have been reported.

Other newly emerging strategies for addressing issues of frail elders are the *bao mu*, eldercare centers, and additional family-oriented policies. The *bao mu* or nursemaid, discussed earlier, offers a low-cost approach to in-home care in urban areas (Ikels, 1990b, p. 234). Eldercare centers are another new approach being developed in two cities in southern China, Guangzhou and Linghai (Ikels, 1990b, p. 240). They are residential facilities for ambulatory elders not needing medical care. In terms of policies oriented specifically toward the family as a source of care, one study (Sankar, 1989, pp. 213-214) describes a new policy directed toward family caregiving of elders: college graduates who are only-children are placed in jobs in the same city in which their parents reside so they will be available as caregivers if or when needed. Recent reports of the state's encouraging widows and widowers to remarry indicate another alternative to long-term care that places emphasis on the family rather than on the state. Begun in the mid-1980s, this approach though not universally accepted, is growing as a practice in urban areas (Ikels, 1990b, p. 238).

CONCLUSIONS

Policies regarding eldercare in the People's Republic of China underwent significant changes during the Communist Party era of Mao and Deng. Despite the long-standing traditional respect for elders that characterizes China's public facade, ample exceptions exist to suggest that other factors influence the daily practices and policies of eldercare. Under the present regime, policies toward population containment, bureaucratic and party reform, and economic reform are having a significant impact on the role and care of the elderly population (Olson, 1988). Together with the growth in the proportion of elderly, these reforms are having an impact on how the society addresses the issues of long-term care and other issues related to an increase in the frail population.

The dominant policy aimed at the growing proportion of frail elders' centers on minimizing the role of the state and constraining the growth of costly medical treatment programs. There continue to be, however, policy suggestions in eldercare that focus on the centrality of the family in partnership with the state. In a symposium on aging held in Beijing in 1989, it was proposed, "While giving full play to the functions of family care for the aged, we should. . . . perfect such care . . . by combining the state, collective, and family. . . . " (Wei & Hu, 1989). This proposal hints at a larger role of the state in the future of eldercare.

Nonetheless, as long as the major responsibility for eldercare is placed on the family, the community, and the work unit, the political system defines the responsibility for frail elders as residing primarily in the social system and, secondarily, as a responsibility of the state-operated medical care system. If so, economic resources can more legitimately be directed toward economic growth and toward increases in the standard of living, especially in urban areas. The policy of reducing the state's burden of the care of elders is reflected in several initiatives now underway: (1) adopting a copayment plan in medical benefit programs; (2) targeting only special elders (the rural childless and urban influentials) for benefits; (3) encouraging family obligations; and (4) encouraging elders to be resources to their families and communities (Ikels, 1990b, pp. 221-222).

Other studies have identified community-level initiatives that illustrate China's emphasis on local or community initiatives in addressing the issues of eldercare. One study (Jia, 1988) gives an example of rural initiatives now underway in China that relieve the state of the economic burden of care for elders. It reports efforts in one village to establish a local pension system for its retirees based on voluntary contributions from workers. Another study (Zhang, 1986) identifies efforts in rural communities to expand local retirement systems for elders, to institute old-age insurance programs, and to promote bank savings for older workers. Where the state does take direct responsibility for eldercare (limited primarily to urban areas), it is largely through increases in the number of hospitals, training of more doctors, a stabilized pension system, and a cost-effective medical insurance program.

The direction of these initiatives remains to be seen, and the decade of the 1990s will reveal more clearly how far the state will shift its policy away from local care of frail elders to a centralized program, and whether the differences in rural and urban long-term care practices will grow or disappear. In addition, the question of the future of state policy is complicated by recent, mounting evidence from research during the last decade that suggests elders still live predominantly with other family members–but the proportion is declining (Goldstein, Ku & Ikels, 1990). Several studies done in both rural and urban settings point to more elders living alone, including one study in a large city in western China, Lanzhou (Yue, 1986), which found that nearly half of the women over age 65 preferred to live separately from their married children. The question is, to what degree, if any, will the increase in independent living contribute to erosion of the family as the principal long-term care unit.

To the degree changes such as those noted above occur in the structure of the family, there will have to be changes in the long-term care practices for frail elders. This does not mean, of course, that there are simple cause-effect relations between family systems and eldercare, but rather that the major social systems and eldercare policy are intricately interconnected. Foremost among those interconnections is the role of the political economy. The complex interrelations among (1) the traditional values of the family, (2) the economic reform programs, (3) the thrust of the political agenda, and (4) the differences between the rural and urban social and economic systems, make prediction difficult. Future eldercare practices will require a careful watch on the family, economy, and political system.

REFERENCES

An, Z. 1982. Reforming the cadre system. *Beijing Review*, 25 (9), 3-4.

Banister, J. (1988). The aging of China's population. *Problems of Communism*, 37, (6), 62-77.

Bianco, L. (1981). Birth control in China: Local data and their reliability. *China Quarterly*, 85, 119-37.

Chen, A. (1970). Family relations in modern China fiction. In M. Freedman (Ed.), *Family and kinship in Chinese society* (pp. 87-120). Palo Alto, CA: Stanford University Press.

Chen, X. (1985). The one-child population policy, modernization, and the extended Chinese family. *Journal of Marriage and the Family, 47*, 193-202.

China News Analysis. (1984). Socialist China, social policy and the elderly. 1257 (March 26), 1-8.

Cowgill, D. (1986). *Aging around the world*. Belmont, CA: Wadsworth.

Davis, D. (1989). Chinese social welfare: policies and outcomes. *China Quarterly, 119*, (September), 577-597.

Davis-Friedmann, D. (1984). The provision of essential services in rural China. In R. Lonsdale (Ed.), *Rural public services* (pp. 5-224). Boulder, CO: Westview Press.

Davis-Friedmann, D. (1985a). Old age security and the one-child campaign. In E. Croll, D. Davin, and P. Kane (Eds.), *China's child family policy* (pp. 149-161). London: Macmillan.

Davis-Friedmann, D. (1985b). Chinese retirement: Policy and practice. *Current Perspectives on Aging and the Life Cycle, 1*, 295-313.

Deng, X. (1983). On the reform of the system of party and state leadership. *Beijing Review, 25*, (9), 3-4.

Ding, H. (1984). Glorious retirement of 813,000 veteran cadres throughout the country. *Chinese Elderly, 11*, 9.

Estes, C., Gerard, L., Zones, J., & Swan, J. (1984). *Political economy, health, and aging*. Boston, MA: Little, Brown.

Goldstein, M., Ku, Y., & Ikels, C. (1990). Household composition of the elderly in two rural villages in the People's Republic of China. *Journal of Cross-Cultural Gerontology, 5*, 1-12.

Henderson, G. (1990). Increased inequality in health care. In D. Davis and E. Vogel (Eds.), *Chinese society on the eve of Tiananmen* (pp. 263-282). Cambridge, MA: The Council on East Asian Studies/Harvard University.

Hu, T. (1984). Health services in the People's Republic of China. In M. Raffel (Ed.), *Comparative health systems* (pp. 141-152). University Park, PA: Pennsylvania State University Press.

Ikels, C. (1990a). Family caregivers and the elderly in China. In D. Biegel and A. Blum, (Eds.), *Aging and caregiving* (pp. 270-284). Beverly Hills, CA: Sage Publications.

Ikels, C. (1990b). New options for the urban elderly. In D. Davis and E. Vogel (Eds.), *Chinese society on the eve of Tiananmen* (pp. 215-242). Cambridge, MA: The Council on East Asian Studies/Harvard University.

Jamison, D., Evans, J., & King, T. (1984). *China: The health sector*. A World Bank Country Study. Washington, D.C.: The World Bank.

Jia, A. (1988). New experiments with elderly care in rural China. *Journal of Cross Cultural Gerontology, 3* (2),139-148.

Kallgren, D. (1985). Politics, welfare, and change: The single-child family in

China. In E. Perry and C. Wong (Eds.), *The political economy of reform in post-Mao China* (pp. 131-156). Cambridge, MA: Harvard University Press.

Liang, J., & Gu, S. (1989). Long-term care for the elderly in China. In T. Schwab (Ed.), *Caring for an aging world: International models for long-term care, financing, and delivery* (pp. 265-287). New York: McGraw-Hill.

Liu, A. (1986). *How China is ruled.* Englewood Cliffs, NJ: Prentice-Hall.

Liu, L. (1990). Social security for state-sector workers in the People's Republic of China: The reform decade and beyond. Unpublished paper.

Liu, W. (Ed.) (1989b). *China social statistics 1986.* Compiled by the State Statistical Bureau of the People's Republic of China. The China Statistics Series. New York: Praeger.

Macciocchi, M. (1972). *Daily life in revolutionary China.* New York: Monthly Review Press.

Myles, J. (1984). *Old age in the welfare state.* Boston, MA: Little, Brown.

Ministry of Public Health. (1986). *1985 Chinese health yearbook.* Beijing: Chinese Health Press.

Oksenberg, M. (1982). Economic policy-making in China: Summer 1981. *China Quarterly, 90,* 165-94.

Olson, P. (1987). A model of eldercare in the People's Republic of China. *International Journal of Aging and Human Development, 24,* 279-300.

Olson, P. (1988). Modernization in the People's Republic of China: The politicization of the elderly. *Sociological Quarterly, 29,* 241-62.

Poston, D., & Gu, B. (1984). Socioeconomic differentials and fertility in the provinces, municipalities and autonomous regions of the People's Republic of China, circa-1982. *Texas Population Research Center Papers.* Series 6: Paper No. 6.011. Austin: University of Texas.

Saith, A. (1981). Economic incentives for the one-child family in rural China. *China Quarterly, 87,* 492-500.

Sankar, A. (1989). Gerontological research in China: The role of anthropological inquiry. *Journal of Cross Cultural Gerontology, 4,* 199-224.

Shehui Baozhang Bao. (1987). [Social Security Newspaper.] Old age homes in China. April 10, 1990, p. 1.

Skocpol, T. (1985). Bringing the state back in: Strategies of analysis in current research. In P. Evans, D. Rueschemeyer, and T. Skocpol (Eds.), *Bringing the state back in* (pp. 3-37). New York: Cambridge University Press.

Social Statistics of China, 1990. (1990) [*Zhongguo shehui tongji ziliao, 1990*]. Guojia tongjiju shehui tongji. Beijing: Zhongguo tongji chubanshe, May.

Treas, J., & Logue, B. (1986). Economic development and the older population. *Population and Development Review, 12* (4), 645-673.

Wei, H., & Hu, R. (1989). *International symposium on aging: Policy issues and future challenges.* Proceedings. Beijing: China National Committee on Aging.

Whyte, M., & Parish, W. (1984). *Urban life in contemporary China.* Chicago, IL: University of Chicago Press.

Wolf, A. (1986). The preeminent role of government intervention in China's family revolution. *Population and Development Review, 12,* (1), 101-116.

Yu, E., Liu, W., Levy, P., & Zhang, M. (1989). Cognitive impairment among elderly adults in Shanghai, China. *Journal of Gerontology: Social Sciences, 44*, (3), S97-106.

Yuan F. (1987). The status and roles of the elderly Chinese in the families and society. *Journal of Beijing University* (Philosophy and Social Sciences) No. 3, 1-8.

Yue, Q. (1986). Family changes and trends in Lanzhou. *Xibei Renkou* [*Northwest Population*], *3*, 8-12.

Zhang, C. (1986). Welfare provisions for the aged in rural China. *Australian Journal of Chinese Affairs, 15*, 113-124.

Zhao, S. (1987). The retirement of veteran cadres in China: Its causes and impact on elderly Chinese. Master's thesis. Kansas City, MO: University of Missouri-Kansas City.

Zhu, C. (1990). Community service with Chinese characteristics–guaranteed community service. Unpublished paper.

The Changing Responsibilities
of the State and Family
Toward Elders in Hong Kong

Nelson Chow, PhD

The University of Hong Kong

SUMMARY. With a predominantly Chinese population and a cultural tradition of respecting the old, Hong Kong has long relied on the family to support its elderly members. Economic success has, however, not spared Hong Kong from encountering the same problems as other industrial societies, such as the loosening of its traditional values. This article examines the changing responsibilities of the state and the family in Hong Kong in supporting the old, and in particular, the effectiveness of the "care in community" policy, which the Hong Kong Government has adopted since the mid-1970s. The examination concludes that the responsibility must now be shared between the state and the family.

Nelson Chow is Professor and Head of the Department of Social Work and Social Administration at the University of Hong Kong. He is specializing in the comparative study of social security systems in East and Southeast Asian countries and has published a book entitled *The Administration and Financing of Social Security in China.*

This article is part of a research project on the support of the elderly in Chinese societies which the author is presently conducting with financial assistance from the Center of Asian Studies, The University of Hong Kong.

[Haworth co-indexing entry note]: "The Changing Responsibilities of the State and Family Toward Elders in Hong Kong," Chow, Nelson. Co-published simultaneously in the *Journal of Aging & Social Policy,* (The Haworth Press, Inc.) Vol. 5, No. 1/2, 1993, pp. 111-126; and: *International Perspectives on State and Family Support for the Elderly* (ed: Scott A. Bass and Robert Morris) The Haworth Press, Inc., 1993, pp. 111-126. Multiple copies of this article/chapter may be purchased from The Haworth Document Delivery Center [1-800-3-HAWORTH; 9:00 a.m. - 5:00 p.m. (EST)].

111

EXISTING POLICIES ON CARE
FOR ELDERS IN HONG KONG

Among countries in the Asian and Pacific region, Hong Kong probably presents itself as the most appropriate example for an examination of the changing responsibilities of the state and the family towards the support of elders. On the one hand, more than 98% of the population in Hong Kong are Chinese, and certain traditional values, such as respecting the old, are often thought to continue to exist in a Chinese society (Ikels, 1983). On the other, economic development in the last 40 years has turned Hong Kong into one of the most affluent cities in East and Southeast Asia. With economic success, it is only natural for one to expect Hong Kong to encounter similar problems as other industrial societies, such as the aging of its population, the weakening of its family system, and the loosening of some of its traditional values (Schulz, 1991). In other words, the Chinese families in Hong Kong may no longer be capable of taking care of their elders as in the past, and there would be a greater pressure on the state to provide the necessary support and care.

To what extent is the above correct? As Hong Kong grows in affluence and becomes completely urbanized, would families there necessarily give less attention to their elders? Could the traditional value of respecting the old co-exist with the modern forces of industrialization and urbanization? If Hong Kong is following in the footsteps of other industrial societies in requiring a greater input from the state in providing care for elders, how should the responsibilities be shared between the state and the family?

The institution of state support for elders has only a short history in Hong Kong. It was in 1973 that a Working Party, set up by the Hong Kong Government to look into the future needs of elders, first acknowledged that there existed in Hong Kong a problem of the aged (Working Party on the Future Needs of the Elderly, 1973). Before that, the government's stand was that the responsibility of caring for elders must fall on the "natural family unit," in particular, the children of the families, and the government must not do anything to "accelerate the breakdown of [this] natural or traditional sense of responsibility" (Hong Kong Government, 1965, p. 5).

This stand was changed in 1977 when the government published a policy paper on the future development of services for elders, which accepted the recommendations of the Working Party (Hong Kong Government, 1977). This change was partly attributed to the growing number of elders in the population, but also and more importantly to the increasing incidence of families failing to meet the needs of their aged members, which was revealed in a survey conducted in 1976 (Hong Kong Council of Social Service/Social Welfare Department, 1978).

The approach to guide the development of social services for elders is officially known in Hong Kong as "care in the community," as it was first used in the Working Party's Services for the Elderly report. As stated in the report, it means that:

> Services should be aimed at enabling the elderly to remain as long as possible as members of the community at large, either living by themselves or with members of their family, rather than at providing the elderly with care in residential institutions outside the community to which they are accustomed. (Working Party on the Future Needs of the Elderly, 1973, p. 15)

When the Working Party made its recommendations, what it had in mind was to minimize the necessity of residential care for elders. Whether or not the Working Party truly believed that the "care in the community" approach was a better form of care would be difficult to tell, but the Working Party frankly admitted that it "looked for solutions which. . . . would cost less, would make least demand on scarce manpower resources and which could be implemented reasonably quickly. . . ." (1973, p. 44). In making its recommendations, the Working Party recognized the fact that the majority of elders in Hong Kong in the early 1970s were living with their families; it thus assumed that this approach "makes the best sense from the point of view of the elderly themselves, their families and the community at large" (1973, p. 15). It concluded that, as long as some care was provided for elders, either by their own families or the community at large, they should be content in the environment they knew.

Since adopting the "care in the community" approach as the guiding principle for the support of elders, a wide range of state community support services including community nursing, home helps, day care, laundry and canteen services, social and recreational activities, hostel accommodation, and respite care have been developed. The supply of these services has, however, always been inadequate; for example, by the end of March 1991, the demand for 30 day care centers for elders has only been met by a provision of nine, and the demand for 30 multi-service centers by a provision of 17 (Social Welfare Department, 1991, Chapter 6). Despite the inadequate supply, the "care in the community" approach was reaffirmed once again in a recent policy paper on social welfare, which states:

> An elderly person should be assisted to live in his own community with dignity and a spectrum of services should be provided in and by the community to facilitate his continued participation in society both socially and, if he likes, economically for as long as possible. (Hong Kong Government, 1991, p. 30)

The "care in the community" approach will thus remain, and although the government is prepared to provide more adequate support for aged members of the society, it also expects the community to continue its caring roles.

In addition to the community support services mentioned above, elders in Hong Kong are also entitled to a number of cash allowances provided by the state. When an elderly person who is a Hong Kong resident reaches the age of 65, he or she can apply for a noncontributory old age allowance. Those between 65 and 69 years have to declare that they have neither an income nor assets above certain prescribed levels to be eligible. When applicants reach the age of 70, no income declaration is required. The amount of the allowance is admittedly insufficient even for a subsistence living and is given as an incentive for the families to take care of their elders. Although the need for retirement pensions has long been established in Hong Kong, relevant schemes on a compulsory basis have yet to be introduced, and elders who fail to make both ends meet can apply for public assistance, which is provided by the state to guarantee everyone in society a basic living standard (Social Welfare Department, 1992). In addition to the various social security payments, the government is also responsible for funding a large part of the community support services mentioned above, although the running of them is often in the hands of nongovernmental organizations. In 1991, the outlay of the government regarding both cash payments and in-kind services for elders, excluding medical care, accounted for about half of the entire welfare budget, or 3% of the total government expenditure.

Family Support and Filial Piety

Before evaluating the "care in the community" approach and its effects on the sharing of responsibilities between the state and the family in supporting the old, it may be necessary to first examine the situation of elders in Hong Kong and the ethical basis upon which this approach has been built. In 1991, the proportion of the population aged 60 and above, who are regarded as old in Hong Kong, stood at 12.8%, as compared to 7.4% in 1971 and 10.3% in 1981. As Hong Kong had by 1991 a total population of over 5.7 million, the number of elders came close to around 730,000. This figure may not seem excessive in comparison with similar ones in most industrial societies, but it is important to note that the aged presently living in Hong Kong are usually migrants, having moved to Hong Kong in the late 1940s and the early 1950s; they are therefore the first generation in Hong Kong to experience aging in a modern industrial society. The environment, and thus the value orientations, within which they now grow old is very different from the one they were familiar with when they were young. This has resulted in a discrepancy between the kind of care they may expect from their families and what their families can actually provide for them (Young, 1990).

In addition to the difference in expectations towards family care, elders in Hong Kong are facing another value conflict in that an increasing proportion of the younger generation, once married, is showing a reluctance to reside with them. The Hong Kong Population Census conducted in 1991 found that "one vertically extended nuclear family," more commonly known as a "three-generation family," accounted for only 10.7% of all households, a decrease from 13.6% in 1981 (Census & Statistics Department, 1991). Other current data sets on elders reveal that about 4% of them are living in various types of institutions, 24% either alone or with another elder, thus leaving about 70% with other members in a family (Central Committee on Services for the Elderly, 1988). Again, when compared with other industrial societies, the percentage of elders in Hong Kong who are residing with their children still appears to be very high, but the trend is definitely on the decline. The noteworthy point is that elders in general still hold it desirable for the children, even after marriage, to reside with their elderly parents, and the increasing trend of the latter moving away is obviously contradictory to the former's beliefs.

The traditional value that has been governing the parent-child relationship among the Chinese is one known as filial piety, which requires the children to show respect for their parents. Although this value has very much been challenged, as Hong Kong is not unlike other industrialized societies, a survey conducted in Hong Kong in 1985 reported that 87.6% of the respondents either agreed or strongly agreed that "the first thing to do in order to build a good society was to have everyone practicing filial piety" (Lau & Kuan, 1988, p. 59). And to fully understand the importance of filial piety, one has to link it up with the significant place occupied by the Chinese family system. In brief, the importance of the Chinese family system comes not only from the functions it performs for its members, but also from the roles it undertakes on behalf of the wider society (Baker, 1979). Hence, within the Chinese family, children are taught not only to respect their parents but also all senior members of society; as Yang once wrote:

> While the functioning of filial piety was limited to relationship between parents and children, their veneration of age was traditionally a means of inspiring respect and obedience by the young toward all the other senior members of the family and society as a whole. (Yang, 1959, p. 51)

Based on the notion of filial piety, a network of relationships is thus established with distinct entitlements and obligations. It is of course difficult to ascertain the extent to which these entitlements and obligations are still valid in present-day Hong Kong but as a value in itself, evidence indicates that it is still very much treasured (Lau,

Lee, Wan, & Wong, 1991). This explains why in the policy paper published in 1991 on social welfare, the Hong Kong Government states: "In Hong Kong it is generally considered a virtue to honor and respect the elderly and it is accepted as a family responsibility to look after the older members as far as possible" (p. 30). The policy that now exists in Hong Kong on care of elders is thus still based on the traditional notion of filial piety, though the government accepts that this notion has been subject to challenges and pressures as the Hong Kong society further develops. As children are believed to be morally obliged to take care of their aged parents, an approach that encourages such practices is perceived to be most appropriate. That accounts for why the "care in the community" approach, first proposed in 1973, has been upheld until today as the guiding principle for the development of social services for elders in Hong Kong.

The "Care in the Community" Approach in Real Perspective

The "care in the community" approach in Hong Kong is not unlike the "open care" or the "community care" model developed in the West (Little, 1982). Conceptually, few can question the general aim of a policy to enable the aged to continue living in the community and maintaining their links with their families and friends. However, as Kathleen Jones, John Brown, and Jonathan Bradshaw point out, "to the politician, 'community care' is a useful piece of rhetoric; to the sociologist, it is a stick to beat institutional care with; to the civil servant, it is a cheap alternative to institutional care . . . " (Jones, Brown, & Bradshaw, 1978, p. 114). Hence, the "community care" approach often promises more than it can actually achieve. This is also true of the situation in Hong Kong.

While the "community care" approach may not necessarily, as argued by Martin Bulmer, "boil down to care by members of the immediate family" (Bulmer, 1987, p. 2), evidence in Hong Kong shows that the family system there does act as the major provider of care for elders. This has been so partly because the majority of elders are still living with their children, but is also due to the fact that the domiciliary services provided by the government are not enough to meet the demand. The burden of supporting the aged falls therefore largely onto the shoulders of the family, and it is no wonder that the "care in the community" approach has sometimes been nicknamed as "care by the community" or even "care by the family."

Other than the need to increase community support services in order to make the "care in the community" approach viable, the approach itself has also been questioned regarding the various assumptions made by the Working Party in 1973. First, as stated in a policy paper on social welfare published by the Hong Kong Government in 1977, the "care in the community" approach could only succeed when the community was a caring one. No elaboration, however, has been given as regards the meaning of a "caring community" except that "these people [the families, neighbors and friends] can do a great deal to sustain the elderly's self respect and social integration and thus to enable the elderly to retain a general sense of satisfaction and fulfillment in the latter period of their lives" (Hong Kong Government, 1977, p. 3). While the contribution of families, neighbors, and friends is not in doubt, more and more people in Hong Kong now are coming to believe that the task of supporting the aged in living a dignified life in the community should fall as much on the state as on families (Law, 1982). The government must therefore work hand in hand with the elders' families, neighbors, and friends in the creation of a "caring community."

Secondly, the "care" that can be provided in and by the community has only been assumed and never clearly defined. It is therefore open to different interpretations. The most common conception is that "care" refers to a whole range of provisions made by the government to meet such basic needs of the aged as those for subsistence, housing, and personal and medical care. Others would have in mind the assistance offered by relatives, neighbors, and friends when elders are sick and weak. Indeed, the "care in the community" approach is so vaguely defined in the Working Party's report, often implying no more than helping elders to remain as members of the community, that it can mean different things to different people.

Thirdly, as mentioned above, when the Working Party put up its recommendation for the adoption of the "care in the community" approach, it was mainly looking for a more cost-effective method of supporting the old. Though this approach cost the government less, families having elders to take care of are bearing the expenses either directly or indirectly. A study on elders awaiting admission into "care and attention homes" in Hong Kong found that the main reason for application into these homes was that most families could no longer afford to have someone staying at home to look after elders; even when they managed to do so, it often implied a sharp reduction in family income as someone would not be able to go out to work (Chow, 1988). From the perspective of family members, the "care in the community" approach is definitely not cost-effective, and means only a shifting of financial responsibility from the state to the family.

In summary, though the "care in the community" approach is found to be ideologically congruent with the notion of filial piety, it suffers nevertheless from a number of shortcomings. First, the burden of care often falls on the family as input from the government, in the form of community support services, is usually inadequate. The "caring community," which is considered to be essential to the implementation of the approach, is often found to be assumed rather than real. And the meaning of "care" is so vague that it is open to interpretation. Finally, it is a heavy financial burden on the family if it has an aged member who needs care.

The Changing Community and the Responsibility of Care

Another theoretical question that the Working Party, in recommending the "care in the community" approach, has not examined in sufficient detail is the definition of "community." When the term was used by the Working Party, it was referred to either as the environment that elders knew, or as sources from which elders could possibly obtain care and attention (1973, p. 15). Hence, the "community" possesses a geographical dimension and at the same time implies a set of social relationships within which help is available. The importance of the "community" is once again stressed in the policy paper on social welfare published in 1991, which states that the well-being of the people ". . . . cannot be achieved without the support of an input from the community through the establishment of networks of informal care and support provided by families, friends and neighbors" (Hong Kong Government, 1991, p. 18). Even if one can accept this understanding of the Working Party on the idea of "community," one has still to ask: What is the geographical boundary of this community? What are the sets of social relationships that do exist to provide elders with care and attention? Does this network of informal care and support exist naturally or has it to be created? What is the relationship between this network of informal support and the system of formal care?

In a report of the Barclay Committee, a committee set up in the United Kingdom in the early 1980s to look at the delivery of personal social work services, "community" was defined as "a network or networks of informal relationships between people connected with each other by kinship, common interests, geographical proximity, friendship, occupation, or the giving and receiving of services for various combinations of these" (Barclay Report, 1982, p. 199). As far as Hong Kong is concerned, the community will probably consist of the networks of relationships established between the aged and other people as a result of kinship, geographical proximity, and the giving and receiving of services. It has been mentioned that the unextended nuclear family in Hong Kong has long been the norm rather than the exception, and that about one in four of elders are either living alone, with another person, or in collective households. Though the majority are still living in a family, and mostly with their children, as the average household size in Hong Kong is at present less than 3.5 persons, the number of family members who are able and willing to help must be very small. In a study on the size of the informal support network, defined as those persons who were ready to offer help, Raymond Ngan found that 13.6% of the elderly respondents had not even one individual, while 58.8% had one to three persons (Ngan, 1990, p. 21). And those ready to help were mostly family members or their immediate kin. In another study on the health situation of elders, Iris Chi and Jik-joen Lee found that less than two persons were ready to offer help to each aged respondent when they were sick or injured, and these again were mostly family members and close relatives (Chi & Lee, 1990, p. 33). Hence, although kinship relationships still form an essential element of the community from which elders can receive care and support, that community is rapidly dwindling in size and is often restricted to one or two immediate family members.

If the community of kinship relationships is diminishing in importance, is there any possibility for it to be compensated for by the relationships established between neighbors, especially when families in Hong Kong are progressively split as a result of internal migration, with young married couples moving to the new towns? Nearly all data available on the degree of neighborliness in Hong Kong, measured in terms of the frequency of contacts between neighbors, indicate that the situation is less than desirable (Chan, 1990). In a study on the lifestyle of the aged in Hong Kong, respondents answered that when they needed help in their daily life, they would first turn to their children (48%), followed by their spouse (24%), and only 11% mentioned their friends and neighbors (Chow & Kwan, 1986, p. 44). More recent studies by Ngan and Sum Young also reported similar results (Ngan, 1990; Young, 1990). This situation is not special to Hong Kong; a national survey of social networks in adult life in the United States in 1980 also found that "82% of the support networks consisted of family members, only 18% consisted of friends" (Antonucci & Akiyama, 1987, p. 523).

One can thus conclude that while neighbors might in future become a more important source of help for elders in Hong Kong, there is little likelihood that they can replace family members. Ideologically, as long as the notion of filial piety still exerts an influence, the obligations of neighbors to help are not as strong as those of family members. There is of course another possibility and that is for the formal care network, comprising the services either provided or financed by the state, to replace the informal care of the family. But as mentioned earlier, the provision of formal care for elders is lagging so far behind demand that only less than 20% of the aged population can have access to such services.

In summary, the "community" that currently exists in Hong Kong as a source of help to the aged comprises mainly the family to which elders belong; neighbors and service networks at best play a supplementary role for a small number of those who either have no family of their own or are fortunate enough to obtain help from their neighbors or social welfare agencies. However, while the family in

Hong Kong still provides a "community" for the majority of the aged, the rapidly decreasing percentage of elders living with their married children implies that the "community," which formulates the basis of the "care in the community" approach, is weakening in strength. Furthermore, it is also difficult nowadays to find relatives to help out. The increasing number of married women employed outside of the family is another phenomenon that has, and will further, weaken the caring function of the family. It can thus be concluded that although the family remains as the most important "community" within which elders can obtain care and support, the extent of help available is both limited and diminishing in scope. On the other hand, there is no sign at the present moment that neighbors and service networks are emerging as viable alternatives.

The Interrelationships Between State and Family Care

As the family still constitutes the most important source of help to the aged, and will continue to do so in many years to come, it is important to further examine the exact nature of care it provides and its relationship with state care. As mentioned before, a compulsory retirement pension scheme is still absent in Hong Kong; as a result, it is not uncommon for elders to turn to their grown-up children for financial support. For those who have no one to support them, their last resort would be to apply for public assistance. At present, about 10% of elders are receiving public assistance. As long as the aged in Hong Kong are not entitled to compulsory retirement pensions, the majority will continue to look to their children for financial support, with a small percentage dependent on public assistance from the state.

Besides financial support, the other forms of care most frequently offered by the family are those connected with daily living activities, such as help with bathing and ambulation. However, it should be noted that the majority of the aged in Hong Kong who live in the community do not actually need a great deal of care from their families. Even for those who are deteriorating in health, representing about 10% to 15% of the total, Chi and Lee found in their 1990 study that the extent of help required was confined to one or two items, usually cleaning and cooking (Chi & Lee, 1990, p. 33). It was also found that those who actually needed help were often the more aged ones of 70 years and above.

Although the number of elders needing personal care is relatively small and consists mainly of the oldest individuals, one has to recognize the fact that family care is diminishing and there is little chance for neighbors to become a viable alternative "caring community." It is therefore necessary for the state to expand its caring roles. In adopting the "care in the community" approach, the Hong Kong Government once committed itself to providing "a range of community services and improved cash benefits that will encourage families to look after their elderly members, or which will enable old people on their own to live independently, and in dignity, in the community for as long as possible" (Hong Kong Government, 1979, p. 14). As discussed earlier, the promise to provide elders with the necessary community support services has not been fulfilled. As a result, many elders living in the community are unable to lead an independent life, not to mention a dignified one. The inadequate provision of community support services has also produced two effects that were unintended when the "care in the community" approach was first proposed. First, as the services are not available to all who need them, they are thus offered to those perceived to be in the greatest need, who often happen to be the frail elders without a family. This situation is not special to Hong Kong. A national study of caregiving for frail elders in the United States reported that "Less than 10% [of caregivers] reported the use of paid services, and those who did rely on formal care were assisting the most severely impaired elders" (Stone, Cafferata, & Sangl, 1987, p. 625). Although the "care in the community" approach in Hong Kong also includes the lonely elders, particularly the frail ones, as its target for assistance, the overconcentration of community support services on this group means that help is scarcely available to families with aged members to care for.

Secondly, as families having aged members to look after often fail to obtain outside support, some inevitably take on the caring task in a negative manner and this has often made elders feel unwanted. Chi and Lee in their study found that elders who required support and care from their families were less satisfied (Chi & Lee, 1989). Young in his study on the dynamics of family care for elders found that the group of older people who were most happy in life were those who could obtain help from both the family and the state (Young, 1990). This is not to imply that families actually make their elders unhappy, but they would certainly find the task much lighter if they could obtain outside help (Kwan, 1991).

This examination of the "care in the community" approach adopted in Hong Kong indicates that, despite the fact that the family system is still the main source of help, there is an increasing demand for formal community support services. So far, the two systems are serving two different target groups of elders and they have yet to truly be integrated with each other. Indeed, it is questionable whether formal and informal support should be identified as two separate systems. Alan Walker once suggested that the rigid division between the formal and informal sectors should be overcome, and that it is better to think more in terms of "social support networks," which "may comprise both formal and informal helps, professional and nonprofessional personnel" (Walker, 1987, p. 381). The recent policy paper of the Hong Kong Government on social welfare also states: "Providing care and support through social networks will be developed and nurtured and it will be necessary to map out the principal objectives and provide supporting services and facilities for the carers involved" (Hong Kong Government, 1991, p. 18).

As the situation in Hong Kong now stands, it will be a long time before the formal and informal sectors can be fully integrated to enable elders to live in the community in dignity. For the majority of them, the family is their most reliable source of help; despite its diminishing functions, it is important to ensure that family members are not overburdened in their task of caring for the aged and hence forced to give it up by institutionalizing them. With the increasing number of private nursing homes, there are already signs that many families are doing exactly this. More adequate provision of formal support services would probably help to relieve the burden on family caregivers; but the help available from friends and neighbors should be further explored. Finally, it should be recognized that filial piety as a value in itself can no longer serve as the prime motivating force for elders to be taken care of in the community. The Hong Kong Government should also no longer be hampered by this ideology, and instead of paying lip service to the need for an active state role, it must now find ways to integrate its efforts with the efforts of families in providing the best care for its aged citizens.

REFERENCES

Antonucci, T.C., & Akiyama, H. (1987). Social networks in adult life and a preliminary examination of the convoy model. *Journals of Gerontology, 42* (5), 519-527.

Baker, H.D.R. (1979). *Chinese family and kinship*. London: Macmillan.

Barclay Report. (1982). *Social workers: Their roles and tasks*. Report of a working party under the chairmanship of Mr. P.M. Barclay. London: Bedford Square Press.

Bulmer, M. (1987). *The social basis of community care*. London: Allen & Unwin.

Census & Statistics Department. (1991). *Hong Kong 1991 population census, summary results*. Hong Kong: Hong Kong Government.

Central Committee on Services for the Elderly. (1988). *Report of the Central Committee on Services for the Elderly*. Hong Kong: Hong Kong Government Printer.

Chen, C.L.W. (1990). Community care in Hong Kong: Questions to be answered. In *Community Development Resource Book 1989-1990* (pp. 25-32). Hong Kong: Hong Kong Council of Social Service.

Chi, I., & Lee, J.J. (1989). *Hong Kong elderly health survey*. Hong Kong: Department of Social Work, University of Hong Kong.

Chow, N.W.S. (1988). *Caregiving for the elderly awaiting admission into care and attention homes*. Hong Kong: Department of Social Work, University of Hong Kong.

Chow, N.W.S., & Kwan, A.Y.H. (1986). *A study of the changing life of the elderly in low-income families in Hong Kong*. Hong Kong: Writers' and Publishers' Cooperative.

Hong Kong Council of Social Service/Social Welfare Department. (1978). *Report of a study on the social service needs of the elderly in Hong Kong*. Hong Kong: Hong Kong Council of Social Service.

Hong Kong Government. (1965). *The aims and policy for social welfare in Hong Kong*. Hong Kong: Hong Kong Government Printer.

Hong Kong Government. (1977). *A programme plan on services for the elderly*. Hong Kong: Hong Kong Government Printer.

Hong Kong Government. (1979). *Social welfare into the 1980s*. Hong Kong: Hong Kong Government Printer.

Hong Kong Government. (1991). *Social welfare into the 1990s and beyond*. Hong Kong: Hong Kong Government Printer.

Ikels, C. (1983). *Aging and adaptation: Chinese in Hong Kong and the United States*. Hamden, CT: Archon Books.

Jones, K., Brown, J., & Bradshaw, J. (1978). *Issues in social policy.* London: Routledge & Kegan Paul.

Kwan, A.Y.H. (1991). *A study of the coping behavior of caregivers in Hong Kong.* Hong Kong: Writers' and Publishers' Cooperative.

Lau, S.K., & Kuan, H.S. (1988). *The ethos of the Hong Kong Chinese.* Hong Kong: The Chinese University Press.

Lau, S.K., Lee, M.K., Wan, P.S., & Wong, S.L. (Eds.). (1991). *Indicators of social development: Hong Kong 1988.* Hong Kong: The Chinese University Press.

Law, C.K. (1982). *Attitudes toward the elderly.* Hong Kong: Department of Social Work, University of Hong Kong.

Little, V.C. (1982). *Open care of the aging.* New York: Springer.

Ngan, R.M.H. (1990). The availability of informal support networks to the Chinese elderly in Hong Kong and implications for practice. *Hong Kong Journal of Gerontology, 4* (2), 19-27.

Schulz, J.H. (1991). *The world ageing situation.* New York: United Nations.

Social Welfare Department. (1991). *The five-year plan for social welfare development in Hong Kong: Review 1991.* Hong Kong: Hong Kong Government Printer.

Stone, R., Cafferata, G.L., & Sangl, J. (1987). Caregivers of the frail elderly: A national profile. *The Gerontologist, 27* (5), 616-626.

Walker, A. (1987). Enlarging the caring capacity of the community: Informal support networks and the welfare state. *International Journal of Health Services, 17* (3), 369-386.

Working Party on the Future Needs of the Elderly. (1973). *Services for the elderly.* Hong Kong: Hong Kong Government Printer.

Yang, C.K. (1959). *The Chinese family in the communist revolution.* Cambridge, MA: Harvard University Press.

Young, S. (1990). The dynamics of family care for the elderly in Hong Kong. Unpublished Ph.D. thesis. Hong Kong: University of Hong Kong.

Under New Management:
The Changing Role of the State in the Care of Older People in the United Kingdom

Alan Walker, DPhil

University of Sheffield, England

SUMMARY. This article examines recent changes and those currently being introduced in the formal care of older people in the
United Kingdom. These are part of a general trend in all welfare
states towards welfare pluralism but, in addition, the United Kingdom represents something of a special case because of the radical
ideological engine that has driven the restructuring of the role of the
state. The first part of the article outlines the main changes–the
promotion of the private sector, the residualization of the public
social services, and the new managerial role of the state in the care of
older people. The second part considers the implications of these
changes for older people and their informal helpers (or caregivers).
The conclusion refers to both the particular changes taking place in
the United Kingdom and, in general terms, to welfare pluralism as a
policy goal.

Alan Walker is Professor of Social Policy and Chairperson of the Department
of Sociological Studies, University of Sheffield, England. He has published
extensively in the fields of social gerontology and social policy, his books including *Ageing and Social Policy* and *The Caring Relationship*. Dr. Walker also chairs
the European Community's Observatory on Ageing and Older People.

[Haworth co-indexing entry note]: "Under New Management: The Changing Role of the State in
the Care of Older People in the United Kingdom," Walker, Alan. Co-published simultaneously in the
Journal of Aging & Social Policy, (The Haworth Press, Inc.) Vol. 5, No. 1/2, 1993, pp. 127-154; and:
International Perspectives on State and Family Support for the Elderly (ed: Scott A. Bass and Robert
Morris) The Haworth Press, Inc., 1993, pp. 127-154. Multiple copies of this article/chapter may be
purchased from The Haworth Document Delivery Center [1-800-3-HAWORTH; 9:00 a.m. - 5:00 p.m.
(EST)].

Social services in all advanced welfare states share at least one thing in common: They are all either in transition or on the verge of transition. It seems that in the organization of social services the only certainties are change and uncertainty. Similar causal factors may also be observed in different societies–socio-demographic change, fiscal austerity, the shift from industrialism to "post-industrialism" or post-modernism, ideological antagonism to state welfare and grassroots pressures–as can their potent conjunction during the late 1980s. Even though the exact combination of these factors and the pace and scale of changes they have produced differs between societies, there is no mistaking the common direction of change, for example, the creation of more mixed economies of welfare, with a diminution of the role of the state and an increase in those of the voluntary and informal sectors; the separation of provider and funding roles; care-packaging, case management; and the tailoring of services to users (Evers, 1991; Friedmann, Gilbert & Sherer, 1987). Because the social services are in a process of flux, it is not possible to say whether or not the changes taking place entail permanent transformations in the welfare roles of the state and other providers. Undoubtedly, though, there are profound realignments underway in the social and economic orders of the advanced industrial societies (Esping-Andersen, 1990; Harvey, 1989), which, in turn, have a deep-seated impact on welfare state regimes of all types. Thus, the purposive attempt by the British government to reconstitute the welfare mix in the social services explicitly called for a "cultural revolution" within the state sector in order for it to adapt to the change in its role from provider to manager.

The first part of this article examines the two main reasons for the changes being wrought in the role of the British state in the provision of social care to older people and other groups and outlines the key features of the changes. The change in ruling ideology represented by the election of the first Thatcher Government in 1979 is identified as the main factor because the policy has been largely a top-down one. However, this policy has articulated some of the grassroots pressures for change in the organization and delivery of the social services that were, slowly and haphazardly, being taken on board in the previous era. Arguably, the United Kingdom represents an extreme case within Western Europe: a long established welfare state that became subject to neo-liberal economic and political management in the late 1970s. This had the effect of accentuating the ideological opposition to the role of the state in welfare, giving it pre-eminence among the various pressures for change. Therefore, the attempt to alter the welfare mix has been more radical than in other Western European countries.

However, at the time of writing, the outcome of the government's far-reaching reforms is not entirely certain because they are being implemented in phases from 1991 to 1993. Although the General Election on April 9, 1992 resulted in the re-election of the Conservative Government pledged to carrying through these reforms, the question as to what resources are available to implement the main phase (from April 1993) has still to be resolved, but meanwhile the government has been severely criticized for underfunding the personal social services (Schorr, 1992). In the second half of the article, the implications of the shifting welfare mix and the changed role of the state are explored, especially their impact on older service users and their informal caregivers.

FROM CONSENSUS TO CONFLICT IN COMMUNITY CARE POLICY

The personal social services (PSS) in Britain are managed and delivered by local government and financed partly by central and partly by local government (whereas the health service comes under the auspices of central government). Provision, including residential care, day care, and home care, goes overwhelmingly to older people (£1,370 million in 1987/88 compared with £180 million to adults with physical disabilities). The policy objective that has dominated discussion in the social services under successive governments over the post-war period is that of community care (Webb & Wistow, 1987, p. 71). Political consensus on this policy objective survived from the 1940s to the 1980s when it underwent a radical transformation. Thus the overriding factor in the active promotion of a shift in the welfare mix in the United Kingdom was the ideological change represented by the election of the first Thatcher government in 1979. A shift in the welfare mix would have taken place without a change of government, for the reasons outlined below, but the Thatcher administration had a decisive impact on the nature, scale, and pace of the shift. Without a radical political agenda behind it, the evolution of alternative welfare mixes would, in all probability, have been as unremarkable as in other European Community countries. Thus, in a nutshell, the gradual evolution of pluralism in the personal social services was overtaken by the Conservative Government's radical political agenda and, in particular, the policy of residualizing public-sector provision.

The post-war party political consensus on community care policy was sustained, in part, by the symbolic nature of the term "community care" and its wide appeal in the policy system. Not surprisingly, the consensus was a precarious one, relying on ambiguity and uncertainty of purpose in policy and the absence of strategic planning; the maintenance of the family, and female kin in particular, as the main providers of care with local social services departments (SSDs) occupying a restricted and junior role; and the subordination of community care services to institutional interests in both the health and social services (Titmuss, 1968; Walker, 1986a). Moreover, community care services were underfunded which, when coupled with the pressures resulting from population ageing, produced a growing "care gap" (Walker, 1985).

Nonetheless, there was a consensus among policymakers on both the secondary role of the formal sector to the informal sector and on the premise that when services were provided *in* the community the most appropriate location for the planning, organization, and delivery of these services was SSDs. This does not mean that local authorities were exclusive providers of social care; there has always been a mixed economy of welfare in this field. But the mixture was very unbalanced, with local SSDs being the dominant providers and the voluntary and private sectors occupying limited roles either independently or, more usually, under contract from SSDs.

So, after 30 years of community care policy, by the late 1970s the burden of care in the informal sector of family, friends, and neighbors was increasing, and institutional budgets continued to dominate both health and social services (Gray, Whelan, & Normand, 1988). Then on to the stage came urgent economic pressures, stemming initially from the fiscal crisis of the mid-1970s but given a particular anti-welfare state slant following the election of the Thatcher government in 1979. These produced severe budgetary and resource constraints and a cost-effectiveness imperative which, in combination with a major expansion in the need for care particularly among very elderly people, created the political will to overcome both the policy inertia and power struggle between sectional interests that laid behind the precarious consensus on community care. But the policy itself departed significantly from the previous consensus. Thus, the emphasis in policy has been purposely shifted away from care *in* the community supported by local authority personnel towards a confusing mixture of care *by* the community itself and private care, regardless of whether in domiciliary or institutional settings.

Signs that the post-war consensus on community care policy was about to be destroyed became apparent soon after the election of the first Thatcher administration. The government's first public expenditure White Paper (Treasury, 1979) combined with a speech by the Secretary of State for Social Services (Jenkin, 1979) marked a radical break with the past–the ending of protected status for personal social services (PSS) spending, the abandonment of the coordination and monitoring of local service provision and the increasing reliance on nonstatutory forms of welfare (Walker, 1986b; Webb & Wistow, 1982)–a trend that was confirmed subsequently by a series of official reports and statements culminating in the National Health Service (NHS) and Community Care Act, 1990. There are three main dimensions to the new policy that unfolded during the 1980s. However, one of them, a radical program of mental health hospital closure, is largely beyond the scope of this article; it concentrates on the other two.

Promoting the Private Sector

While the primary intention of social services policy during the 1980s and early 1990s appears to have been the negative one of reducing the role of local authorities in the provision of care, the 1980s also witnessed for the first time the active official encouragement of the private sector. This new policy direction was signaled early on in the life of the first Thatcher government when, soon after coming to power, the Department of Health and Social Security (DHSS)[1] began to encourage a switch in the provision of residential care from the public sector to the private sector.

It did so, first of all, by reducing the resources available to local authorities, by 4.7% in 1979/80 and 6.7% in 1980/81 (Walker, 1986b, p. 17). Secondly, while the public sector received the stick, the private sector was given the carrot. The DHSS agreed not only to meet the full cost of care in private residential and nursing homes for those on income support (the scheme providing minimum guaranteed resources) but it also allowed local offices to set limits on such board and lodging payments as were deemed appropriate for their area. As a result, the number of places in private residential homes for older people and people with physical and mental disabilities nearly doubled (increased 97%) between 1979 and 1984, and, by 1990 had risen by 130% since 1979. The parallel story of expenditure on both residential and nursing homes was that of a rapid increase from £6 million in 1978, to £460 million in 1988 and to £2.3 billion in 1991. The proportion of people in private residential homes receiving help with their fees through income support payments increased from 14% in 1979, to 35% in 1984 and, by 1991 had reached 70% (Bradshaw & Gibbs, 1988, p. 4; NACAB, 1991, p. 6).

Since this growth in spending conflicted with the government's policy of reducing public expenditure, the DHSS acted to stem the flow of resources first by freezing local limits in September 1984 and then, in April 1985, by imposing national limits for board and lodging payments. These limits, at the time of writing are £150 for residential and £200 for nursing homes for older people and £175 and £215 respectively for homes for people with mental disabilities and, therefore, still represent a major source of income to the private sector.

Residualizing the Social Services

A series of what seemed as they occurred to be separate policy developments over the past 13 years may, with the benefit of hindsight, be seen as part of an evolving government strategy aimed at turning local authority SSDs from the main providers of formal care into something far more limited: the provider of those residual services that no one else could or would take on.

In 1980, in a speech to directors of social services departments, the then Secretary of State, Patrick Jenkin, outlined a supportive and decidedly residual role for the social services: "a long-stop for the very special needs going beyond the range of voluntary services" (Jenkin, 1980). In 1981, the White Paper on services for older people asserted, in a widely quoted phrase, "care in the community must increasingly mean care *by* the community" (DHSS, 1981, p. 3). The previous year Jenkin had justified the cuts in PSS expenditure and the closure of long-stay hospitals on the unsubstantiated assumption that the informal and voluntary sectors would expand.

But it was Jenkin's successor as Secretary of State, Norman Fowler, in a 1984 speech, who provided the clearest and most detailed outline of the new residual role proposed for social services. The fundamental role of the state, according to Fowler, was "to back up and develop the assistance which is given by private and voluntary support" (Fowler, 1984, p. 13).

In 1986, the Audit Commission–the body responsible for auditing local government expenditure–proposed various organizational changes aimed primarily at clarifying the overlapping responsibilities of health and social services authorities. In response to the debate following the Audit Commission report, Sir Roy Griffiths (director of a large supermarket chain) was appointed in March 1987 to examine community care arrangements particularly with regard to older people. The report of the Griffiths inquiry was published in March 1988, the White Paper, *Caring for People,* followed in November 1989 and, within days, the NHS and Community Care Bill was published. Together, these policy developments suggest a strategy aimed at residualizing the social services. This strategy has three elements.

In the first place, the provision of community care is being deliberately *fragmented.* Though sometimes presented blandly as promoting a more mixed economy of welfare, the main motivations here have been to curtail the monopoly role of local authorities in the delivery of formal care–an aim that, as we shall see, has already been achieved in several parts of the country with regard to the residential care of older people–and to encourage the growth of cheaper sources of informal and quasi-formal care. Sir Kenneth Stowe, the former permanent secretary of the DHSS, described this new approach as "letting a hundred flowers bloom."

Second, there is *marketization.* As we have seen, while finances for local authority services have been tightly controlled, the private sector has been encouraged to expand by the open-ended provision of social security board and lodging subsidies. Contracting out, or purchase of service contracting, has a long history in the personal social services but it has been used primarily in relation to the voluntary sector (Webb & Wistow, 1987, p. 89). So far, direct privatization has not affected the social services to the same extent as the NHS. But the Local Government Act 1988 gave the Secretary of State for the Environment powers to add to the list of services that must be contracted out.

Third, the government has pursued a twin-track policy of *decentralizing* administration and operations, while *centralizing* control over resources. This is one manifestation of the broader New Right strategy of rolling back the frontiers of the state while centralizing state control (Gamble, 1987). In theory, the decentralization of operations offers the prospect of greater user involvement in service management and delivery. But this is unlikely to be realized unless resources and responsibility are also devolved.

The cumulative impact of these three sets of policy developments is a strategy aimed at further residualizing the role of local authorities providing community care (for a similar conclusion concerning the Netherlands and a contrast with Sweden, see Baldock & Evers, 1990).

Although some aspects of these policies were to be found under former governments, a concerted strategy of this sort has not been identifiable previously. Of course in relation to the totality of care, both formal and informal, the social services have never been anything other than residual. The essence of the Thatcher and Major governments' approach towards community care, however, is that they are attempting, with some success, to reduce the role of local authorities as providers *within* the formal sector. Furthermore, it is intended to fill this artificially created care gap with a mixture of private, voluntary, and informal care.

Grassroots Pressures

While the post-war period up to the end of the 1970s may have been characterized by policy consensus among politicians, the users of the social services were increasingly dissenting. Disillusionment with certain aspects of the social services set in gradually and, during the 1980s became more and more outspoken. The residualization policy has articulated some of the criticisms of the social services and has, thereby, gained some legitimacy from them. There are four sorts of criticism (for a full account, see Walker, 1987).

First, more and more users of the social services have been complaining about their bureaucratic organization, complexity, and lack of responsiveness to felt needs (Fisher, 1989; Mayer & Timms, 1970; Sainsbury, 1980). Some groups of users–such as people with disabilities–have formed self-advocacy movements to press their case for greater influence over their own lives and the services they use.

Second, there is the distinct feminist critique of the gendered nature of care that has developed since the late 1970s into a devastating indictment of both informal and formal care. Feminists have been primarily responsible for demonstrating that community care is, in fact, mainly care by female kin and also that care consists of two dimensions: labor and love (Finch & Groves, 1980; Land, 1978; Walker, 1981). This has led to a demand for alternative approaches that do not exploit women (Dalley, 1983; Finch, 1984; Waerness, 1986). Of course this criticism is of direct relevance to a discussion of shifts in the welfare mix because the policy of residualization makes assumptions about the availability of female labor to provide informal care. Furthermore, many innovations in social care rely on the unpaid or low paid services of women and, therefore, they may be subjected to the same feminist critique as traditional social services.

Third, out of this feminist critique has come a specific case mounted by those people responsible for providing informal care. During the 1980s, caregivers began to form self-help and pressure groups to support themselves and represent their views. Together with researchers they have shown that community care policies have paid very little attention to the needs of caregivers and the state has done very little to support the activities of the six million informal caregivers (Oliver, 1983; Wright, 1986).

Fourthly, users and caregivers from ethnic minority groups have begun to criticize the social services for failing to recognize both their specific needs and the extent to which their cultural background and their experience of racism should be reflected in service provision (Atkin, 1991).

These four criticisms have contributed to a disillusionment with social services and, in combination with demographic and economic factors that are common to all welfare state societies, have created significant pressures for change in the organization and delivery of services. But it is the political ideology of the present government and its predecessors that have dictated the scope of the changes that are taking place in the welfare mix. The strategy is residualization but the rhetoric takes the form of increasing choice and flexibility. So far the major shift in the welfare mix has taken place in the residential sector and by increasing the burdens on families, but the proposals currently being implemented are intended to transform the division of labor within the formal sector.

The New Managerial Role of the Local State

The NHS and Community Care Act represented the culmination of the previous decade of policy, as outlined above, and established a new framework for services. The Act was based on the White Paper *Caring for People* (DH, 1989) which, in turn, was derived in large measure from the recommendations of the Griffiths Report (1988). The Act received the royal assent on June 29, 1990 and was due to be implemented in full on April 1, 1991. However, on July 18, 1990 the Secretary of State announced a delay in the implementation of the main financial provisions of the Act until April 1993. It would appear that the government was rather nervous about the implications of the changes for local tax levels (Henwood, Jowell, & Wistow, 1991).

What are the main changes in policy that will flow from the implementation of the Act? The White Paper defined four key components of community care which together reflected the emphasis on promoting choice in policy developments over the previous decade;

they were cast in the language of consumerism as well. They are: services that respond flexibly and sensitively to the needs of individuals and their caregivers; services that intervene no more than is necessary to foster independence; services that allow a range of options for consumers; and services that concentrate on those with the greatest needs (DH, 1989, p. 5). In the White Paper, "choice" is defined as "giving people a greater individual say in how they live their lives and the services they need to help them" (DH, 1989, p. 4). This is to be achieved in two main ways: a comprehensive process of assessment and care (or case) management, which "where possible should induce [the] active participation of the individual and his or her carer," and a more diverse range of nonstatutory providers among whose benefits is held to be "a wider range of choice of services for the consumer" (DH, 1989, pp. 19, 22).

The main policy changes are as follows: local authorities become responsible as "lead agencies" for assessing individual need, designing care arrangements, and insuring that services are delivered. Thus, crucially, the provision of services is separated from their purchase, and it is expected that SSDs will make maximum use of private and voluntary services. Local authorities are to produce and publish plans for the development of community care services. A new funding structure will be established for those with public support in nonstatutory residential and nursing homes (though the changes do not apply to those in residence up to April 1993). Resources are to come from a single unified budget, in the hands of local authorities, comprising existing social services resources *plus* the care element of social security board and lodging allowances deemed likely to be necessary by the government for new users.

Some controversy surrounded the award of lead agency status to SSDs following the publication of the Griffiths Report. It was conjectured that the report's release on the day after the 1988 Budget and the long delayed response to it signalled the government's displeasure with this central recommendation. On the face of it, too, this proposal (now enacted) is completely at odds with the residualization strategy described earlier. However, Griffiths made a clear distinction between responsibility for insuring that care is provided and actual provision: "[T]he role of the public sector is essentially to ensure that care is provided. How it is provided is an important but secondary consideration" (Griffiths, 1988, p. vii). This places the Griffiths Report, White Paper, and 1990 Act firmly in the mainstream of government policy stretching back to 1979. The role established for local authorities covers the management and regulation of care, *not* its provision. It is this change that has been referred to as requiring a cultural revolution among service providers in the public sector. As managing agents, they will oversee the further residualization of public sector provision while encouraging the expansion of the private and voluntary sectors.

IMPLICATIONS OF THE SHIFTING WELFARE MIX

What are the likely implications for older service users, potential users, and their informal helpers of these radical developments in the organization and delivery of services? Again, since the main changes in the mix of service provision for older people and people with disabilities have not yet been implemented, what follows is to some extent speculation. There are five main sets of issues to be considered, and they are presented here as dichotomies in order to emphasize the dilemmas and conflicts underlying policy in this field even though this format runs the risk of oversimplification.

Need and Choice versus the Market

As we have seen, so far at least the most visible shift in the welfare mix has been within the residential sector of care for older people. Over the decade 1979-1989, the numbers of beds in the private residential sector trebled, to 31.1 places per 1,000 people over 65. Yet it is estimated in the United Kingdom that only 11 places per 1,000 people over the age of 65 are required to support severely disabled older people. Thus a significant proportion of older people in private residential homes, perhaps as much as one half, do not need to occupy residential places on the basis of disability. The implications of this development for the social status and citizenship of older people are profound. For example, substantial numbers of them are entering residential homes because there is no reliable community-based alternative and no funding for them to buy their own. As a result this group prematurely encounters the dependency-creating aspects of residential regimes (Walker, 1982). Moreover, the rapid expansion of the private sector has been skewed towards the younger age groups of older people where need is less than among the very elderly. For instance, between 1979 and 1989 there was a 38% growth in the numbers aged 85 and older and this was accompanied by a 12% rise in the number of private residential beds; yet while the population aged 65 to 74 declined by 9%, there was a 15% growth in private provision for this group. In other words, the uncontrolled expansion of the private sector militated against the distribution of services according to need.

Some policy analysts (see, for example, Day & Klein, 1987) have taken the view that the growth of the private sector of residential care is beneficial because it increases choice in an expanding "mixed economy of welfare." Indeed, the appeal to increased choice has proved an important source of popular legitimation for the fast expansion of the private sector. However, while it is true that there has been a rapid multiplication of private homes, as a result of the government's residualization strategy, local authority residential places have been cut for all age groups of older people, especially those aged 85 and older, and the building of sheltered housing for older people has fallen sharply. Yet genuine choice requires a range of alternative forms of care: public-sector homes, sheltered housing, day care, the opportunity to remain in an ordinary dwelling with community support. But, ironically, this sort of choice has been severely restricted by the "perverse incentive" (Audit Commission, 1986) for older people to enter residential care created by social security payments. Furthermore, when it comes to entering a residential home the concept of "choice" is rarely appropriate. The need for residential care usually arises because of a crisis of care in the informal sector, leaving little time to "shop around" for alternatives. Thus, as Jonathan Bradshaw (1988) has confirmed, the promise of choice held out by the supporters of the private sector is often illusory.

There is a growing body of evidence that the creation of a large private residential care sector has not resulted in greater choice for older people as the protagonists of this policy had claimed. For example, a study of the private sector by the Centre for Policy on Ageing found that only a quarter of residents exercised any choice about the home they were admitted to, while nearly a quarter said that their admission resulted from unsolicited arrangements by a third party (Bradshaw, 1988, p. 18). Choice between private homes is severely restricted by factors such as geographical location, waiting lists, and ability to pay. There is, for example, a clear north-south divide in the public/private mix of welfare. Private nursing home beds in the South West outnumber those in the Northern region by seven times. In two regions, South East and South West Thames, the private sector was providing more than half the total beds for older people by the mid-1980s (Larder, Day & Klein, 1986).

Within local areas choice can be restricted by the admissions criteria applied by private homes, often excluding confused or demented people or those who are difficult to control. Thus there is a tendency for private homes to select or "cream off" the less severely disabled older people, leaving the more severely disabled for the public sector (ADSS, 1986; Audit Commission, 1992). Also, private homes often levy charges above the income support limits, requiring top-up payments from older people or their relatives, or they make supplementary charges for single rooms or items such as laundry. This problem worsened after the government imposed national limits on board and lodging payments in 1985 and then failed to raise the benefit ceilings in line with increases in residential and nursing home charges. As a consequence and despite the high cost of these payments to the Exchequer, more and more older residents found their benefits inadequate to cover the fees charged. According to August 1988 DSS figures (the latest at the time of writing), 42% of private residents receiving income support were paying fees above the national limits (Social Services Committee, 1990).

The research evidence also suggests that residents are not able to exercise much choice once they are inside private homes. A study of homes in North Yorkshire found that 21% had undergone a change of ownership in the previous 18 months (Bradshaw, 1988, p. 19). Residents have no say in such changes and are not always informed before they happen, nor do they have any choice about other changes in the character of their home:

> Residents entering small homely homes may find them enlarged. Residents have no control over the mix of residents or who shares their bedroom. As charges move ahead of (income support) limits residents may find themselves shifted into double or treble rooms, required to commit their pocket money to supplement the (income support) allowance or being subsidized by relatives–often without their knowledge. (Bradshaw, 1988, p. 19-20)

Questions have been raised not only about the distributional consequences of the government's policy of promoting the private sector, considerable doubts have also been raised about the quality of the care provided in a minority of homes. As the private residential sector mushroomed, evidence mounted of abuse, misuse of drugs, and other forms of restraint, fraud, lack of hygiene, and fire hazards in some homes (Counsel and Care, 1992; Harman & Lowe, 1986; Holmes & Johnson, 1988).

So far this discussion has concentrated on private care from the perspective of service users, partly in order to dispel the myth that an extension of the private market must, by definition, enlarge choice. But, while the quality of care is substandard in some private homes, there is also plenty of evidence to show that the pay and conditions for staff working in some of them are well below their public counterparts. There are documented examples, too, of untrained and low-paid staff having to bear high levels of responsibility for the care of vulnerable people and being threatened with dismissal if they join a trades union (Holmes & Johnson, 1988, pp. 82-105).

It is sometimes argued that a reduced role in the provision of public services could be balanced by an increased regulatory role for the state (Day & Klein, 1987). Indeed, this is one of the intentions behind the changes currently being implemented. However, the regulatory regime is relatively weak and there are insufficient resources to provide for effective inspection. This is partly because the ideological driving force behind the expansion of the private sector is wary of over-regulation, in case it hinders the efficient operation of the market. In addition, there is the fact that the rapid growth of the private sector has created a vociferous lobby which is resisting the granting of far-reaching regulatory powers to inspection units.

The implementation of the NHS and Community Care Act is likely to further constrain choice. As a result of the ideological context of these changes, a premium is placed on nonstate forms of provision. So, local authorities will be expected to employ competitive tendering or other means of marketing the production of welfare. This gives a rather biased meaning to the "mixed economy of care." For example, the White Paper suggested that one of the ways in which social services departments could promote a mixed economy of care is by "determining clear specifications of service requirements, and arrangements for tenders and contracts" (DH, 1989, p. 23). But evidence from the United States indicates that competitive tendering may actually *reduce* the choice available by driving small producers out of contention (Demone & Gibelman, 1989). This is likely to effect specialist provision for some minority group needs, such as those for older ethnic minorities and particular disability groups.

Consumerism versus Empowerment

Despite the political rhetoric concerning user involvement accompanying the White Paper, neither the Act nor the policy guidelines arising from it contain any concrete proposals for user involvement or empowerment. In the absence of clear guidelines for such involvement, it is likely that professional opinions will continue to dominate. This is evident to some extent in the language employed in the White Paper: "managers of care packages," "case managers," and "caring *for* people." Thus, rather than determining their own packages of care, service users are apparently still seen as passive receivers of care. The situation is similar regarding the prominence given to care (or case) management, which can be either administration centered or user centered. In the context of the pre-eminence given to the goals of value for money and economic efficiency, case management is likely to prove to be primarily an administrative tool for cost containment.

Thus, when viewed from the perspective of service users, the conception of user involvement underlying the proposed cultural revolution is a very restricted one based on a simplistic market analogy (Walker, 1991a, 1992). The Griffiths Report, White Paper, and NHS and Community Care Act all derive from the limited form of supermarket-style consumerism which assumes that, if there is a choice between "products," service users will automatically have the power of exit from a particular product or market. Of course even if this is true in markets for consumer goods, in the field of social care many older people are mentally disabled, frail, and vulnerable; they are not in a position to shop around and have no realistic prospect of exit.

Underlying the consumerist model of social care are two questionable assumptions. It is assumed that monopolies only operate in the public sector. Also it is assumed that the private sector can adequately substitute for the public sector. But, as far as, for example, an older person currently resident in either a public *or* a private home is concerned, her provider *is* the monopoly power because she has no alternative. Having a range of theoretical alternatives will not make the consumer sovereign if she cannot exercise effective choice. Moreover, a financial transaction does not necessarily mean the bestowal on the purchaser of either influence or control over the provider. Furthermore, unlike markets for consumer durables, in the field of social care if the private producer goes out of business this will not only have immense human consequences but the public sector will be expected to pick up the pieces. In other words, the private sector exercises equivalent power over users to public providers but it does not necessarily carry the same responsibility.

The only way that frail and vulnerable service users can be assured of influence and power over service provision is if they or their advocates are guaranteed a voice in the organization and management of services. This would, in turn, ensure that services actually reflected their needs. In practice, the weak form of consumer consultation being pursued in Britain currently under the 1990 Act could consist of no more than an occasional survey among users together with minimal individual consultation at the point of assessment. Thus, despite the rhetoric concerning "packages of care," a cultural revolution, and making services more responsive to users, in practice the government's proposals are silent on how user involvement can be ensured and, in fact, are characterized by old-style paternalism.

In contrast to the consumer-oriented model, the user-centered or empowerment approach would aim to involve users in the development, management, and operation of services as well as in the assessment of need. The intention would be to provide users and potential users with a range of realizable opportunities to define their own needs and the sort of services they require to meet them. Both caregivers and care recipients would be regarded as potential service users. Where necessary, the interests of older people with mental disabilities would be represented by independent advocates. Services would be organized to respect users' rights to self-determination, normalization, and dignity. They would be distributed as a matter of right rather than discretion, with independent inspection and appeals procedures, and would be subject to democratic oversight and accountability.

This distinction between the two ideal types of consumerism and empowerment reflects a philosophical dichotomy between the repression and the liberation of individual consciousness. This dichotomy transcends the more familiar one between individualism and collectivism by recognizing that *both* privately and publicly organized systems of care may reject user involvement and limit the power of users. Of course philosophy is important, but what really counts in the current era of cost effectiveness are the financial consequences resulting from a particular policy. For example, SSDs have long provided direct payments to enable people with disabilities to buy their own services such as home helpers or occupational therapists. A study conducted in 1990 found that 59% of SSDs made such payments either directly or through intermediaries such as housing associations (Hatchett, 1991). These payments represent a model of a truly flexible service–taking welfare pluralism beyond a narrow focus on choice between formal and quasi-formal providers toward genuine user power. But such payments are actually illegal under the 1948 National Assistance Act, which forbids local authorities to make cash payment in lieu of services. If the government had wanted to extend flexibility and user empowerment, it could have taken the opportunity provided by the 1990 Act to legalize these payments. It not only declined to do so but went so far as to defeat a House of Lords amendment to the Parliamentary Bill designed to make the payments legal. The main reasons appear to be the government's fears concerning the financial implications of providing an open-ended commitment to pay cash to people in need of services and their caregivers and that the payments would be demanded as a right.

Rights versus Discretion

The professed aim of the new policy to increase choice and sensitivity to user requirements is likely to be compromised by the process of assessment, which is inevitably required to ration resources. Thus no one is to receive public funding for residential care after April 1993 unless they have been assessed and recommended by case managers. This process is bound to limit individual choice and user influence while, conversely, enhancing the power of bureau professionals. Moreover, users do not have a right to elect to be assessed and there are no safeguards–such as an appeals procedure–for those who disagree with professional assessments.

The distribution of the PSS in the United Kingdom has never been based on legally enforceable rights. The only rights in this field have been granted through the social security system; for example, the attendance allowance, intended to allow people with disabilities, including older people, to buy their own home care; the invalid care allowance, a small payment to those giving up work to care for a disabled relative; and payments for those entering private homes. But even the limited right to social security board and lodging payments that older people have in order to enter private residential homes will be replaced by care management discretion. Moreover, when coupled with the parallel changes taking place within the NHS, there is a clear danger that hospital care which is free at the point of use will be replaced by discretionary social care which may also have charges levied on it. Thus, alongside the expansion in private residential and nursing homes, there has been a decline in the average length of stay for older people in geriatric wards (from 77.5 days in 1979 to 44.8 days in 1986) and it is increasingly common for older people to move directly from hospital to nursing homes. Moreover, as noted earlier, the NHS has already begun to radically reduce its continuing care facilities for older people in anticipation of the changes in community care services to be implemented in 1993. These developments also serve to remind us that welfare pluralism should not be confined to a simple state/nonstate dichotomy; welfare may derive from different sources *within* the state. Thus in the past bureau-professionals in the health service and personal social services have often vied competitively for control over the welfare of older people. Now, because the private sector is the only one expanding in line with or ahead of need, medical consultants are able to bypass social service staff and arrange a direct transfer from hospital to private home. The new community care system will put a brake on this exercise of professional power and therefore may result in conflict between the health and social services.

The shift within the welfare mix from public to private and voluntary provision also affects citizenship rights in other ways. For example, lines of accountability become less straightforward. Who is responsible: the service provider, the case manager, or the local councillor? The increasing prominence given to equal opportunities policies will be diminished in significance by the atomization of care provision under a cost-effectiveness imperative. Similarly, the option of choosing public provision instead of private or voluntary care will be closed off.

Universalism versus Innovation

The government's fragmentation strategy has resulted in financial support being given to a range of promotive voluntary schemes designed to fill gaps in existing provision or demonstrate the effectiveness of a particular innovation. Examples include day centers, caregivers' relief schemes such as the Crossroads Care Attendant Scheme, and the payment of small sums of money to voluntary home caregivers. At the same time, many local authorities are carrying out experimentation and innovation without government support either because there are no funds available or the project runs counter to the government's ideology, or both. Also there are a number of high profile schemes aimed at organizing packages of care in a more responsive way than under standard social services. The best known of these are the Kent Community Care Scheme, the Dinnington project and the Neighbourhood Support Units initiative (Bayley et al., 1981; Challis & Davies, 1986; MacDonald, Qureshi, & Walker, 1984; Warren & Walker, 1992). Major new initiatives are occurring with great regularity, the latest of which–Elderly People's Integrated Care System–is based on the Californian ON LOK model and is attempting to provide a fully integrated health and social services system. Such innovations, notably the Kent Community Care Scheme, have shown that it is possible to provide home care to people who would normally have been in residential care and at an average cost that is lower than that of a residential home.

However, while there are many positive features of the experiments in community care, a word of caution is necessary. By definition, the process of pluralistic service innovation has been haphazard and confined to very small local areas and, therefore, it has tended to reinforce territorial disparities in social services. The process of innovation has also reflected the political color of local authorities and the desire of the government to sponsor particular kinds of change. This raises a fundamental issue of human rights. These sorts of innovations were not sought by the people concerned, nor did they have an equal voice to that of the service providers in the process of innovation–they are top-down innovations–though, of course, the honorable motives of those responsible for these new developments are not in doubt. In addition, the result of fragmentary innovation is that people with similar needs in different parts of the country, or sometimes local area, are experiencing very different forms of care, based on different assumptions, sorts of providers, and, crucially, rights of access. Older people and other groups of people with disabilities are, in effect, being used as guinea pigs in the testing of service innovations.

This is an issue that those who argue against universalism must confront. At the same time it must be acknowledged that the universalism associated with the UK model of PSS is a very minimal one indeed and one that is characterized by territorial injustice in the formal sector and over-reliance on the family and especially female kin (Bebbington et al., 1990). Thus, as noted earlier, long-term underfunding has created a growing care gap, with the result that most older (and younger) people with disabilities do not receive sufficient assistance to cover all of their care needs and many receive none at all. Moreover, there is no evidence of a wide dissemination of innovative approaches, such as paying neighbors for care, which instead remain largely confined to the demonstration projects. Yet these projects are sometimes used as examples of how the welfare mix has changed.

In the social security field, the most noteworthy innovation in recent years was the creation of the Independent Living Fund in 1988. This is a small fund (originally £5 million but raised to £20 million in 1990) which currently helps some 7,000 severely disabled people to live in the community by granting them one-off or regular payments, sometimes as much as £300 per week. However, people with disabilities have no statutory rights to money from the fund and no right of appeal if requests are refused. In effect, the fund is a hybrid form of state-backed charity. Not surprisingly, organizations representing disabled people have argued that the fund should become part of the social security system and extended to help more of the six million people with disabilities in the United Kingdom, the vast majority of whom are over 65.

The Family versus Community Care

Despite the rhetoric concerning the needs of caregivers, there are no proposals designed to ensure that their needs are taken into account. In the absence of such guarantees, of course, there is a danger that, under financial pressure, they will be downplayed. Furthermore, the fact that there might be a conflict of interest between caregivers and care recipients is not recognized by the government's proposals. But this is a very real problem facing older people, their caregivers, and service providers. The failure to address this dilemma stems from the assumption underlying both the White Paper and the Griffiths Report that the family should in all circumstances be the primary source of care. However, research has shown that this confidence in familism is sometimes misplaced: family care can be both the best *and* the worst form of support (Qureshi & Walker, 1989). It is at its worst when it is imposed on a relationship that has been antagonistic for many years. This can lead to resentment on the part of caregivers and provide a basis for potential abuse of the older person. If policymakers continue to assume that the family is always the soundest basis for care, they will overlook existing conflicts in the caring relationship and be guilty of imposing some potentially destructive relationships on both caregivers and care recipients.

This highlights an inherent conflict between the family and the state in the care of older people and others with disabilities. There does *not* have to be a conflict between caregivers and care recipients as some have suggested (Finch, 1984) though, of course, the provision of care is often based on conflictual gender relations within the nuclear family. As far as the family is concerned, *both* caregivers and care recipients have an interest in social care that prevents dependency and does not overburden female kin. This would promote harmonious intergenerational and gender relations. But for its part the state seeks to maintain the primacy of the family in the provision of care and also a minimalistic system of social care. The main mechanisms for achieving these goals are familism at an ideological level and underfunding on the ground (Walker, 1991b). The only Western countries that appear to be near to overcoming this conflict between state and people are the Scandinavian ones, where the goal of gender equality in the labor market is coupled with the relatively generous funding of support services. Appositely, those countries have been described as "women friendly" (Balbo, 1987).

In the United Kingdom and other liberal welfare states, the desire to maintain the primacy of the family in the care of its dependents also contributes to the masking of the productive contribution of mainly female caregivers and the maintenance of the distinctions between paid work and productivity and unpaid work and unproductive activity. Of course unpaid nonmarket work is a key element of the infrastructure that supports both the wage system and the welfare system in advanced industrial societies. It is likely that shifts in the welfare mix will perpetuate the exclusion of informal caregivers from the public recognition and respect (and pay) received by formal caregivers because, in the United Kingdom at least, these changes are driven by the search for cheaper nonstate forms of care rather than by a desire to improve the quantity and quality of support available to older people and their informal caregivers.

CONCLUSION

Two sets of conclusions may be drawn from this analysis: one concerning the likely outcomes of the particular changes taking place in the United Kingdom and the other concerning the general application of welfare pluralism as a goal of social services reform.

Social services provision in the United Kingdom for older people and other people with disabilities is minimalistic and therefore overreliant on unpaid female labor. Principally under the steam of neo-liberal ideology, the welfare mix has been shifted dramatically in one sector in the direction of private provision. Proposals to transform the role of the public sector–from provider to "enabler"– are in the pipeline and these have been extensively trailed by government ministers over the last four years. Public-service providers have been exhorted to take part in the cultural revolution required to achieve the intended change. So far it appears that the hearts and minds of these providers have not followed the government's lead– the cultural revolution has not occurred. This is due to a combination of factors: chronic underfunding, worries about the quality of care provided by the private and voluntary sectors, suspicions about government motives, and the desire to remain as providers and not be confined to a largely managerial role. In this sort of adverse context, it is difficult to see how choice can be increased and users and caregivers can be empowered.

In the United Kingdom, therefore, debate about market choice and pluralism has diverted attention from discussion of the *nature* of the services themselves, be they public, private, or voluntary. For example, are services intended to prevent dependency or merely to care for the dependent? Should they be dominated by providers or users? Should they be rigid or flexible? The creation of a more flexible, user-empowering system of services calls for a cultural revolution of a different sort–one aimed at changing working practices *within* the dominant public sector in order to forge a partnership with older service users. Of all the European Community countries, Denmark is closest to this goal because it has the most extensive infrastructure of services to build on (Walker, 1992), whereas in the United Kingdom services are stretched very thinly, which means that even when public-sector staff want to work in more flexible ways they are usually swamped with work and therefore lack the space to think and operate more flexibly (Allen, Hogg, & Peace, 1992).

Welfare pluralism is not a panacea for the universal problem of care provision for the growing populations of older people, unless the policy goal is the narrow one of exit. If the aims are service quality, prevention of disability and caregiver breakdown, and providing older users with a genuine voice, policymakers should focus first on changing the state sector–the dominant one in the majority of European countries–rather than concentrating the bulk of their efforts on the search for cheaper alternatives.

NOTE

1. The DHSS was split into two departments on July 25, 1988: Health (DH) and Social Security (DSS).

REFERENCES

Association of Directors of Social Services. (1986). *Who goes where?* London: Author.

Allen, I., Hogg, D., & Peace, S. (1992). *Elderly people: Choice participation and satisfaction.* London: Policy Studies Institute.

Atkin, K. (1991). Health, illness, disability and black minorities: A speculative critique of present day discourse. *Disability, Handicap and Society,* (1), 37-47.

Audit Commission for Local Authorities in London and Wales. (1986). *Making a reality of community care.* London: Policy Studies Institute.

Audit Commission for Local Authorities in London and Wales. (1992). *The Community Revolution.* London: Her Majesty's Stationery Office.

Balbo, L. (1987). Crazy quilts: Rethinking the welfare debate from a woman's point of view. In A. Showstack Sassoon (Ed.), *Women and the State* (pp. 45-71). London: Hutchinson.

Baldock, J., & Evers, A. (1990). Emerging new forms of social service provision: The examples of innovations in the care of the elderly in the Netherlands, Sweden and the United Kingdom. Paper presented to the XII World Congress of Sociology, Madrid, July.

Bayley, M., Parker, P., Seyd, R., & Tennant, A. (1980). *The Dinnington project.* Sheffield, England: University of Sheffield.

Bebbington, A., Davies, B., Baines, B., Charnley, H., Ferlie, E., Hughes, M., & Twigg, J. (1990). *Resources, needs and outcomes.* Aldershot, England: Gower.

Bradshaw, J. (1988). Financing private care for the elderly. York, England: Department of Social Policy and Social Work: University of York.

Bradshaw, J., & Gibbs, I. (1988). *Public support for private residential care.* Aldershot, England: Avebury.

Challis, D., & Davies, B. (1986). *Case management in community care.* Aldershot, England: Gower.

Counsel and Care (1992). *What if they hurt themselves?* London: Counsel and Care.

Dalley, G. (1983). Ideologies of care: A feminist contribution to the debate. *Critical Social Policy, 8,* 72-81.

Day, P., & Klein, R. (1987). The business of welfare. *New Society,* June 19, 11-13.

Demone, H., & Gibelman, M. (1989). *Services for sale: Purchasing health and human services.* London: Rutgers University Press.

Department of Health, U.K. (1989). *Caring for people,* Cm 849. London: Her Majesty's Stationery Office.

Department of Health and Social Services, U.K. (1981). *Growing older,* Cmnd 8173. London: Her Majesty's Stationery Office.

Esping-Andersen, G. (1990). *The three worlds of welfare capitalism.* Oxford: Polity Press.

Evers, A. (1991). Introduction. In J. Kraan, B. Baldock, A. Davies, L. Evers et al., (Eds.), *Care for the elderly–Significant innovations in three European countries* (pp. 1-6). Frankfurt: Campus/Westview.

Finch, J. (1984). Community care: Developing non-sexist alternatives. *Critical Social Policy, 9,* 6-18.

Finch, J., & Groves, D. (1980). Community care and the family: A case for equal opportunities? *Journal of Social Policy, 9* (4), 487-514.

Fisher, M. (1989). (Ed.) *Client studies.* Sheffield, England: Joint Unit for Social Services Research.

Fowler, N. (1984). *Speech to Joint Social Services Annual Conference,* September 27. London: Department of Health and Human Services.

Friedmann, R., Gilbert, N., & Sherer, M. (1987). (Eds.). *Modern welfare states.* Hemel Hempstead, England: Wheatsheaf.

Gamble, A. (1987). *The free economy and the strong state.* London: Pluto.

Gray, A.M., Whelan, A., & Normand, C. (1988). *Care in the community: A study of services and costs in six districts.* York, England: Centre for Health Economics, University of York.

Griffiths, Sir R. (1988). *Community care: Agenda for action.* London: Her Majesty's Stationery Office.

Harman, H., & Lowe, M. (1986). *No place like home.* London: House of Commons.

Harvey, D. (1989). *The condition of postmodernity.* Oxford: Blackwell.

Hatchett, W. (1991). Cash on delivery? *Community Care*, May 30, pp.14-15.
Henwood, M., Jowell, T., & Wistow, G. (1991). *All things come (to those who wait?)*. London: Kings Fund Institute.
Holmes, B., & Johnson, A. (1988). *Cold comfort*. London: Souvenir Press.
Jenkin, P. (1979). *Speech to Social Services Conference*, Bournemouth, England, November 21.
Jenkin, P. (1980). *Speech to the Conference of the Association of Directors of Social Services*, September 19.
Land, H. (1978). Who cares for the family? *Journal of Social Policy, 7* (3), 357-84.
Larder, D., Day, P., & Klein, R. (1986). *Institutional care of the elderly: The geographical distribution of the public/private mix in England*. Bath, England: University of Bath.
MacDonald, R., Qureshi, H., & Walker, A. (1984). Sheffield shows the way. *Community Care*, October 18, 28-30.
Mayer, J., & Timms, N. (1970). *The client speaks*. London: Routledge.
National Association of Citizens Advice Bureaux. (1991). *Beyond the limit*. London: Author.
Oliver, J. (1983). The caring wife. In J. Finch and D. Groves (Eds.), *A labour of love?* (pp. 72-78). London: Routledge.
Qureshi, H., & Walker, A. (1989). *The caring relationship*. London: Macmillan.
Sainsbury, E. (1980). Client need, social work method and agency function: A research perspective. *Social Work Service, 23*, 9-15.
Schorr, A. (1992). *The Personal Social Services: An outside view*, York, England: Joseph Rowntree Foundation.
Social Services Committee (1990). *Community care: Future funding of private and voluntary residential care*, HC 257. London: Her Majesty's Stationery Office.
Titmuss, R.M. (1968). *Commitment to welfare*. London: Allen & Unwin.
Treasury (1979). *The government's Expenditure Plans 1980/81*, Cmnd 7746. London: Her Majesty's Stationery Office.
Waerness, K. (1986). Informal and formal care in old age? Paper presented to the XIth World Congress of Sociology, New Delhi.
Walker, A. (1993). Towards a European agenda in home care for older people: Convergencies and controversies. In A. Evers and G. van der Zanden (Eds.), *Better care for dependent people living at home: Meeting the new agenda in services for the elderly*. Netherlands Institute of Gerontology.
Walker, A. (1991a). Increasing user involvement in the social services. In T. Arie (Ed.), *Recent advances in psychogeriatrics 2*. London: Churchill Livingstone.
Walker, A. (1991b). The relationship between the family and the state in the care of older people. *Canadian Journal on Aging, 10* (2), 94-112.
Walker, A. (1987). Enlarging the caring capacity of the family: Informal support networks and the welfare state. *International Journal of Health Services, 11* (4), 369-386.
Walker, A. (1986a). Community care: Fact and fiction. In Willmott, P. (Ed.), *The debate about community* (pp. 4-15). London: Policy Studies Institute.

Walker, A. (1986b). More ebbs than flows. *Social Services Insight*, March 29, pp. 16-17.

Walker, A. (1985). *The care gap*. London: Local Government Information Service.

Walker, A. (1982). Dependency and old age. *Social Policy and Administration, 16* (2), 115-35.

Walker, A. (1981). Community care and the elderly in Great Britain: Theory and practice. *International Journal of Health Services, 11* (4), 541-557.

Warren, L., & Walker, A. (1992). Neighbourhood support units: A new approach to the care of older people. In F. Laczko and C. Victor (Eds.), *Social policy and elderly people* (pp. 74-95). Aldershot, England: Avebury.

Webb, A., & Wistow, G. (1982). The Personal Social Services: Incrementalism, expediency or systematic social planning? In A. Walker (Ed.), *Public expenditure and social policy* (pp. 137-164). London: Heinemann.

Webb, A., & Wistow, G. (1987). *Social work, social care and social planning: The Personal Social Services since Seebohm*. London: Longman.

Wright, F. (1986). *Left to care alone*. Aldershot, England: Gower.

Eldercare Policy Between
the State and Family:
Austria

Josef Hörl, Univ. Doz. Dr.

University of Vienna, Austria

SUMMARY. Certain aspects of the Austrian system of social security and public welfare for the elderly, on the one hand, and family caregiving, on the other hand, are reviewed. In 1993, a new attendance allowance act for needy persons is being introduced in Austria. This reform includes cash payments on seven different levels according to the degree of need and is supposed to increase the opportunity of choice for the elderly. This assumption remains dubious; it should not be expected that a significant number of new informal caregivers can be recruited. Furthermore, empirical evidence shows that the elderly themselves clearly prefer the expansion of social services over paid family caregiving. There is a need for more research regarding the effects of interaction among the elderly, the family, and professional caregivers and for the promotion of an empowerment approach.

Josef Hörl is Associate Professor of Sociology and Social Gerontology at the Institute of Sociology, University of Vienna.

[Haworth co-indexing entry note]: "Eldercare Policy Between the State and Family: Austria," Hörl, Josef. Co-published simultaneously in the *Journal of Aging & Social Policy*, (The Haworth Press, Inc.) Vol. 5, No. 1/2, 1993, pp. 155-168; and: *International Perspectives on State and Family Support for the Elderly* (ed: Scott A. Bass and Robert Morris) The Haworth Press, Inc., 1993, pp. 155-168. Multiple copies of this article/chapter may be purchased from The Haworth Document Delivery Center {1-800-3-HAWORTH; 9:00 a.m. - 5:00 p.m. (EST)].

155

THE AUSTRIAN SOCIAL SECURITY SYSTEM

Basic Features

The social security system in Austria has two major components: social insurance and social assistance. While social insurance is mainly financed by earnings-related contributions shared between the insured and employers, and to a smaller and varying degree, by central government subsidies, social assistance is financed from general taxation.

Social insurance is the most important program in the Austrian social security system; 99% of the population is enrolled in one or more subsections of this system. It is responsible for more than nine tenths of total social expenditures; the proportion that social assistance represents of total expenditures on social security has somewhat gone up in the last few years. One of the reasons for this is the increasing cost of care for very old and/or dependent persons. Currently, about 1% of the GDP or 4% of all social expenditures are spent for (nonmedical) care (Steiner, 1992).

Under the constitution, both legislation for social insurance and its implementation are federal responsibilities. The social insurance institutions are formal, autonomous self-governing bodies, although their respective status is subject to control by the central government authorities.

The basis for Austrian social policy was established in the late 19th century. Only a very gradual development took place, originally excluding the elderly from social security. Social insurance in general has been compulsory since 1955. As late as 1970, a pension insurance scheme was introduced covering farmers (Weigel & Amann, 1987).

Legislation in social assistance progressed even more slowly. By constitutional law, responsibility for social assistance matters comes within the competence of the nine Austrian provinces. It must be underlined that the elderly are not entitled as a right to benefits under social assistance legislation.

On the one hand, the social assistance organizations of the provinces fulfill certain special tasks such as the maintenance and running of various social services while, on the other hand, they take over responsibility where the social security network leaves gaps:

the costs of rehabilitation for older persons no longer gainfully employed are, for example, borne by the local social assistance authorities.

A notable feature of social assistance activities at provincial and community levels is the close cooperation between the provincial and local institutions, and nongovernmental, private, and charitable organizations. These latter organizations have been entrusted through legal contracts with a number of tasks in the field of social services (Badelt & Pazourek, 1991).

Summarizing, life in Austria is safeguarded by a comprehensive and complex system of social security and public welfare. At the same time, political power of the elderly remains weak. At present, there is neither an official national statement of rights for the elderly nor a central government bureau for the elderly. Pensioners' organizations are closely affiliated to political parties. They make public announcements on concrete problems and are active in commenting on legislative initiatives in matters of the aged population. However, they do not possess any formal right of veto and cannot be considered as an important lobbying force.

Economic Security

Post-war economic stability has been guaranteed by the two most influential power groups, employers and employees. In Austria, their cooperation has become institutionalized within a system called a "social partnership." It is designed to keep in check the development of wages and prices by close cooperation between these interest groups. They exercise influence on issues far beyond labor relations, for example, on retirement, pension, and caring issues.

The financial situation of the elderly has become quite secure, making them independent from family support. Principally, old-age pensions are calculated on the basis of the length of the insurance period and the average gross earnings over the "best" 15 years of work life. If the old-age pension is below a legally prescribed minimum, the difference is paid in the form of supplementary benefits, so-called compensation allowances. This "minimum pension" is fixed annually; in 1992, the minimum amounted to ATS 6,500 (or $690) per month for a single person. Eleven percent of all male and 17.5% of all female pensioners (24% of all widow pensioners) received such a minimum pension (as of December 1991). In addition, there are a number of other benefits available for older persons with low incomes, such as exemption from payments for telephone and radio/television, reduced fares on public transport, and so forth.

Health Care Services

Health insurance covers practically the entire population. A large proportion of public health expenditures is spent by the provinces and communities, especially on the construction of hospitals and on operating costs not reimbursed by health insurance institutes. Hospital care is in principle free of charge for all insured persons. Health insurance also covers treatment by doctors, medicines, and medical aids. Treatment by a doctor is free of charge if he or she is under contract to the health insurance institute. Since 1992, professional qualified home nursing is covered by the health insurance system in order to lessen the burden resting on hospitals and nursing homes, that is, to postpone or shorten hospitalization periods.

About 20% of all Austrians aged 80 and older are accommodated to some sort of institution. This is a ratio of 4.5 nursing beds and 6.5 beds in residential homes for 100 Austrians above 75 years (Steiner, 1992). These figures must be regarded as rather low by international standards. The regional variation according to size is high; for instance, the largest single nursing home complex (in Vienna) accommodates no less than 3,000 old people.

Supportive Services for the Elderly

Legal definitions for social services and retirement and nursing homes as well as the range of existing services vary greatly between the provinces. To a certain extent this is justified since, apart from Vienna and a couple of other larger cities, Austria still is a country of small communities. To give just two remarkable examples: in rural Burgenland, Austria's easternmost province, there is a service called "institutionalized neighborhood help." The volunteering neighbor takes on the responsibility for the care of an elderly person in the neighborhood. She or he is supervised by a social worker and gets a more or less symbolic payment by the provincial government.

In Vorarlberg, Austria's westernmost province, another unique and unconventional form of care can be found: mutual associations to provide home care for the sick and old on a purely private basis. Through this decentralized system, about one third of the province's population has an immediate right to be supported by a professional nurse in coordination with family lay care (Fülöp, Schäfer, & Frisch, 1988).

In all provinces, social services for the elderly are a major social assistance benefit. They cover all domestic health services, assistance in running the household, services for improving social contacts, recreation schemes, and homes for the aged. Both in terms of scope and organization, home help services are the most extensively developed services in the field of care of the elderly; 2.1% of all Austrians aged 65 and older receive these services.

In some remote areas, however, home help is still practically nonexistent. In Vienna, on the other hand, there has been an eightfold increase in home help caring hours since the early 1970s. Of course, the importance of social services is especially marked for the very old; in Vienna, social services are the main source of support for a quarter of all persons in need over 70 years but only for less than 10% of the persons in need under 70 years.

CONCEPTS OF STRENGTHENING INFORMAL CAREGIVING

The rapid expansion of organized services within the last decades in most industrialized countries (Riede, Schott-Winterer, & Woller, 1988) is symptomatic of social changes. We should be aware of the decreasing *relative* importance of families for the basic needs of the aged. The development towards increased utilization of formal sources of support does not mean that family and kinship are becoming unimportant or only suppliers of affection. Informal care exceeds formal care even in the most advanced welfare states. But we should be warned not to over-idealize and overburden family support networks with expectations that cannot be fulfilled.

Neglecting this, the fiscal crisis of the welfare state and a certain conservative backlash in ideology have led some policymakers to recommend a strengthening of family solidarity and even a more or less pronounced "re-privatization" of support tasks.

In particular, the idea that families need to be strengthened has resulted in the question as to whether it would be desirable and efficient to pay volunteers or family caregivers. This approach gathered momentum and is now considered a serious option in numerous European countries as well as in the United States (Evers, Pijl, & Ungerson, 1992; Linsk, Keigher, & Osterbusch, 1988), because the concepts of care, based on paid professional help, have proved too expensive from a financial point of view. Costs have increased much more than the service volume, due to higher quality standards, improved staffing, better wages, and reduced working hours. Expansion of professional help is impracticable from a labor market point of view, too, regarding the restricted pool of nursing and social personnel.

From a financial point of view, there are two main concepts of strengthening informal care: first, direct payment for care through care allowances for family help; second, indirect payment through attendance allowances for dependent persons to be used by them for remunerating formal and informal help and care. Other measures, like social security benefits and tax deductions for carers, are playing a minor role, at least in Europe.

THE AUSTRIAN SYSTEM
OF ATTENDANCE ALLOWANCE

In Austria, there exists a traditional type of attendance allowance for pensioners, called *Hilflosenzuschuss* (helpless benefit). Currently (as of December 1991), about 15% of all pensioners receive this benefit. There has been a significant rise–in fact, a doubling–in the number of recipients since the 1970s, reflecting mainly the sharp increase in the number of the very old. The median attendance allowance amounts to approximately ATS 2,900 or $260 per month (as of 1991). The amount of the allowance is *not further differentiated* according to the degree of need. Although the attendance allowance is, in principle, not restricted to the elderly, more than 90% of the recipients are 60 years or older, the majority of them being in their eighties or nineties.

The official goal of the attendance allowance, as defined by social insurance law, is to cover the additional expenditures resulting from helplessness and need of care. It is required that the pensioner must be helpless and dependent from other persons, that is, he or she must be in permanent need of help and attendance. Considerable variations in awarding this allowance exist between the different social insurance institutions. For example, former miners and farmers but also blue-collar workers (and their widows) are awarded the attendance allowance much more frequently than former employees. It is not clear at all whether these marked differences reflect true differences in grades of helplessness and caring necessities between the occupational groups or reflect divergent screening procedures and–at least to some extent–are the result of the wish to compensate partly low pension incomes.

Unfortunately, there is no systematic evidence of how the money from attendance allowances is actually spent. Scattered impressions indicate quite clearly that the attendance allowance is regarded by the elderly as an integral part of their pension payment and is not perceived as money dedicated specifically to purchase medical aids and caregiving services from whomsoever. Of course, many older people do give money generously to their offspring and sometimes also to other people but there seems to be no "cash nexus" (Sundström, 1986) between attendance allowances and financial donations to relatives or other informal helpers, on the one hand, and the receiving of supportive services, on the other.

The Reform Act of 1993

A major federal reform of the attendance allowance (renamed *Pflegegeld*) will be implemented in 1993. The allowance will still be paid directly to the indigent person, independent of the reason for the handicap and the means of the person. As an important new feature, the attendance allowance would be provided at seven different rates according to the degree of need, which is determined by both medical criteria and by the extent to which a person's capacity to live independently is reduced. The minimum payment from this new attendance allowance is proposed to be about ATS 2,500 (or $230) per month; the maximum payment could be as high as ATS 20,000 (or $1,800) for severely handicapped persons needing, for example, permanent infusions or artificial respiration devices. Recipients of the former *Hilflosenzuschuss* will automatically be classified at the second lowest level (ATS 3,600, or $330).

It is assumed that the provision of an increased cash payment should promote the opportunity of choice for the potential client. Notwithstanding official statements, the reform is targeted toward encouragement of family and other informal service networks. There is also the tacit assumption that eventually a market for social and health services will develop. Furthermore, an agreement will be necessary between federal and provincial agencies to secure a minimum supply of social services and nursing homes throughout the country.

DISCUSSION

The efficiency of this reform act remains doubtful. On the one hand, the reformed allowance probably will accomplish improved social equity by allocating payments strictly on the basis of a comprehensive and detailed *need* assessment; even more important, the needy elderly will be entitled as a *right* to these benefits. On the other hand, the proposed range of choice alternatives is only theoretical. Recent survey results (Hörl, 1993) show that even among *current* family caregivers a majority rejects the idea of a payment for a family care scheme; instead, they favor social service expansion. It is very unlikely that *new* family carers or new volunteers can be recruited through a system of economic remuneration like this one. It is even less likely that women will give up full-time paid employment for badly paid caregiving labor. So the attendance allowance will function primarily as a matter of social justice, a sort of premium for rewarding persons fulfilling the norm of filial responsibility, that is, the proportion of the costs borne by those already committed may be somewhat lessened. If the provision of incentives would simply supplant existing efforts and do little to change the minds of those who do not now provide care to do so, the policymakers' intentions will fail to mitigate the fiscal consequences of a trend toward reduced family efforts.

The services of private-market organizations are expensive and used only by a wealthy minority. They play only a marginal role in the whole Austrian care market (Badelt & Pazourek, 1991). There will simply not be enough money available from attendance allowances to develop a well-functioning market.

The proposed agreement between federal and provincial authorities to guarantee a minimum supply of social services and nursing homes is merely a declaration of intent. It will be–as until now–restricted by scarce funds and labor shortages and cannot be financed through contributions from the elderly's attendance allowances.

Furthermore, with total client discretion over funds, there is no way to protect the client's interests or handle her or his administrative tasks. There are plans to implement some kind of quality control with regard to services. This is primarily conceived as a precautionary measure against the abuse of the elderly by unscrupulous private suppliers. Supervision of public service providers will take place only by intra-organizational controlling. There are no feasible control mechanisms imaginable at all to evaluate the quality of family caregiving. Many frail and vulnerable elderly in their eighties or nineties are not in a position to "shop around" as most consumers do. Consequently, the opportunity of choice will be on paper only. In all probability, attendance allowances: (1) will go either to family members already providing care, (2) will serve as cost-contributions for conventional social services, or (3) will not be spent at all for caring purposes, because of lack of available local services or a string of other possible reasons. Of course, the third option is completely unsatisfactory from an equity point of view.

It must be also taken into consideration that the health care system often enough functions in complete isolation from the social services. Problems of coordination will become even more complicated in the future when the elderly client will get "free" medical treatment as usual by doctors and home nurses but will be required to "purchase" social services by means of his or her attendance allowance.

Last but not least, as Gordon Streib (1990) and Pamela Doty (1986) have pointed out, complex assessment problems will arise. There will be periodic monitoring required to determine whether the older person should be granted a continued attendance allowance. Direct payments should also be made only to those elderly who are mentally competent to handle their own finances. But what kinds of mental disability should disqualify elderly persons from managing the allowance by themselves–only severe cases of dementia, or also cases of emotional disturbances or depression? Ethical questions arise, such as whether relatives (who may have strong vested interests) should be eligible to handle the finances or whether the elderly should be assisted by a neutral guardian who will act for them under consideration of the degree of their disablement. The various investigative procedures would certainly be costly and perhaps inefficient. In consequence of such experiences, comparable programs in Sweden were dismantled during the 1980s (Sundström, 1986).

Empirical Evidence

Empirical research among the urban elderly shows a clear preference for the further expansion of social services and not for payments for private, informal care. In Vienna, 61% declare themselves for the further expansion of services; only 39% prefer payment for informal care (Hörl, 1992a; for similar Norwegian and United States results, cf. Daatland, 1990; Doty, 1986).

It is striking that results show no significant difference between elderly respondents who declare to be in need for help and those who do not; both groups vote clearly in favor of more social services. The expressed preference for social services is especially strong among those older persons already benefitting from such help.

On the other side, elderly currently receiving help from kin are somewhat less strongly convinced that social services should get top priority in the future. Obviously, they want their current carers to benefit from such a paid family caregiving program. Yet, still only about half of this group has a preference for the option of paid private care.

In the same way, elderly who rate themselves as physically handicapped are more inclined to prefer the public financial support of private carers; however, even among the most disabled group there is a fifty-fifty situation, not a clear-cut priority for paid family caregiving.

Finally, it must be stressed that those elderly preferring social services over paid family caregiving are well integrated into family networks and definitely not cut off from contacts with their children. These respondents have close and frequent contacts with their children, as far as personal visits and telephone calls are concerned.

What explanations can be offered for the clear preference of a further expansion of social services versus paid family caregiving?

As has been mentioned before, the social-service sector has experienced tremendous growth. It is kind of a post-war success story. In the wider public, and especially among the elderly, social services are already regarded as a traditional and reliable way of retaining independence in daily life. Despite this, only a small minority of the elderly people in Austria actually receive regular assistance by home help. The reluctance to use formal support does not prevent attitudinal acceptance of services: "the stigma connected to the client status has more or less disappeared" (Daatland, 1990).

On the other side, the concept of paid family caregiving seems to be looked upon as a strange idea. Direct and official payments for a caring relationship between, let's say, mother and daughter, still are regarded as contradictory to the very idea of family. Family caregiving is still motivated primarily by three factors: love and affection, a sense of gratitude, and societal norms of spousal or filial responsibility (Hörl, 1989).

This is true even if actually there are considerable financial flows from the old to the young. Yet, one has to bear in mind that these flows are not so-to-speak "cash on delivery of service," but normally take rather tortuous paths, as "gift relationships" (Titmuss, 1970), for example, in the form of presents to grandchildren, singular contributions to buy a house or a new car, legacies, and so forth.

The elderly consider affectional ties with their children more important than tangible services and, consequently, they are reluctant to "overstrain" family nursing resources. There appears to be a pronounced tendency by the elderly to deny filial obligation toward old parents in the case of long-term care. The attitude that they should not burden their own children with their more severe personal difficulties probably reflects a fear that this might precipitate other problems. And it is not unreasonable to expect that regular payments for family care could create a string of unforeseen psychological and practical difficulties.

The long-standing formula of "intimacy at a distance" has been verified many times (Rosenmayr, 1990); it reflects the wish to be "somehow" close, for practical and emotional reasons for support on both sides; and yet–also on both sides–to remain separate, for reasons of autonomy and in order to "domesticate" dependencies. Obviously, intergenerational households are regarded as a potential source of conflict. One might say that "intimacy at a distance" is characteristic of intergenerational relationships in Western societies. The final result of paid family caregiving, however, might easily force generations into undesired closeness. Obviously, such a development is rather feared than wished.

CONCLUSIONS FOR FAMILY AND SOCIAL POLICY

Relations between the elderly and their families in industrialized societies can only be understood and analyzed when taking into consideration the intervention of the welfare state.

It must be remembered, however, that there are two target populations in caregiving policy: the elderly and their families. The elderly, due to their vulnerability to chronic disability, have one set of needs. Their families, engaged in the process of helping the older relative, have needs specific to the supportive role they have undertaken. The needs of each population may not always coincide; for example, personal sacrifices in the process of helping may eventually lead to the exhaustion of family support and demand the introduction of social services.

In view of the experiences with attendance allowances until now and the highly skeptical attitudes toward payment of family carers, it is not expected that a cash grant program (under whatever legal title) will successfully bridge the rationality of bureaucratic organizations with the norms and emotional bonding found in family and kin networks, as Marvin Sussman (1985) has argued.

Cash payment is no truly innovative form of care. A user-centered or empowerment approach (Bond, 1992; Walker, 1992) would have to involve users and formal and informal caregivers in the development, management, and operation of services as well as in the assessment of need. Balancing the needs of providers and recipients within service-oriented programs would have also the advantage of providing help in targeting special needs groups. For example, problems resulting from depression or dementia cannot be tackled adequately by cash grants.

At the moment, there exists very little coordination or cooperation among the elderly, their families, and social services. Family members are hardly involved in the planning and monitoring of service delivery to their elderly relative; for example, a recent panel study has shown that even nine months after the beginning of social service one third of family caregivers had not made the acquaintance of the home help. There is "co-existence" but no "joint venture." Frequently, however, staff members are successful in modifying official rules to a great extent, although the bureaucratic environment allows the development of intimacy and love only within rather strictly defined limits (Hörl, 1992b).

The administrators should give more attention to such interactive processes. The value of the low-tech worker is underestimated (Morris, 1989). It is not self-evident that highly efficient delivery of services is best suited to serve the needs of recipients. In fact, the more services are performed in a swift and smooth way, the more disturbing and stressful for the client they may prove. In the future, we will have to deal with the problem of how to translate such knowledge into specific programs and social policies.

REFERENCES

Badelt, Ch., & Pazourek, J. (1991). Care for the elderly in Austria. In A. Evers, & I. Svetlik (Eds.), *New welfare mixes in care for the elderly* (vol. 2) (pp. 13-33). Vienna: European Centre for Social Welfare Policy and Research.

Bond, J. (1992). The politics of caregiving: The professionalization of informal care. *Ageing and Society, 12*, 5-21.

Daatland, S.O. (1990). 'What are families for?': On family solidarity and preference for help. *Ageing and Society, 10*, 1-15.

Doty, P. (1986). Family care of the elderly: The role of public policy. *The Milbank Quarterly, 64*, 34-75.

Evers, A., Pijl, M.A., & Ungerson, C. (1992). Payment for care. International research project. *Eurosocial Newsletter*, No. 59/60, 25-27.

Fülöp, G., Schäfer, E., & Frisch, R. (1988). *Hauskrankenpflege in Österreich.* Vienna: Österr. Bundesinstitut für Gesundheitswesen.

Hörl, J. (1989). Looking back to caregiving. *Journal of Cross-Cultural Gerontology, 4*, 245-256.

Hörl, J. (1992a). Paid family caregiving: An alternative to social services? Paper presented at the intercongress meeting of the RC #11 of the International Association of Sociology, Stockholm, June 24-26.

Hörl, J. (1992b). *Lebensführung im Alter. Zwischen Familie und sozialen Dienstleistungen.* Wiesbaden: Quelle & Meyer.

Hörl, J. (1993). Familiale Betreuung von Müttern und Schweigermüttern. Unpublished research paper.

Linsk, N.L., Keigher, S.M., & Osterbusch, S.E. (1988). States' policies regarding paid family caregiving. *The Gerontologist, 28,* 204-212.

Morris, R. (1989). Challenges of aging in tomorrow's world: Will gerontology grow, stagnate, or change? *The Gerontologist, 29,* 494-501.

Riede, Th., Schott-Winterer, A., & Woller, A. (1988). Soziale Dienstleistungen und Wohlfahrtsstaat. *Soziale Welt,* 39, 292-314.

Rosenmayr, L. (1990). *Die Kräfte des Alters.* Vienna: Atelier.

Steiner, H. (1992). Zur Versorgung hilfs- und pflegebedürftiger Menschen in Österreich. In Bundesministerium für Arbeit und Soziales (Ed.), *Bericht über die soziale Lage* (pp. 129-146). Vienna: Bundesministerium für Arbeit und Soziales.

Streib, G.F. (1990). The family, the polity, and the life course. Paper presented at the XIIth World Congress of Sociology, Madrid, Spain, July 9-13.

Sundström, G. (1986). Family and state: Recent trends in the care of the aged in Sweden. *Ageing and Society,* 6, 169-196.

Sussman, M.B. (1985). The family life of old people. In R.H. Binstock, & E. Shanas (Eds.), *Handbook of aging and the social sciences* (2nd ed.) (pp. 415-449). New York: Van Nostrand Reinhold.

Titmuss, R.M. (1970). *The gift relationship.* London: George Allen & Unwin.

Walker, A. (1992). Towards a European agenda in home care for older people: Convergencies and controversies. In A. Evers & G. van der Zanden (Eds.), *Better care for dependent people living at home* (pp. 1-37). Nijmegen: Institute of Gerontology/European Centre for Social Welfare Policy and Research.

Weigel, W., & Amann, A. (1987). Austria. In P. Flora (Ed.), *Growth to limits. The Western European welfare states since World War II* (pp. 529-609). Berlin: Walter de Gruyter.

The Evolution of the System of Care for the Aged in Denmark

Dena Shenk, PhD

University of North Carolina at Charlotte

Kitter Christiansen, MA

Løkken, Denmark

SUMMARY. In Denmark, formal services are viewed as a *right* to be used by any member of that society who is in need of assistance, premised upon a societal model of mutual self-help. The focus here is on the dual themes of philosophical consistency and of transition in the formal system of services and delivery of care in Denmark. Denmark's system centers on meeting the basic needs of the elderly while enabling individuals to retain control over decisions regarding their own lives. It was effective during the economically expansive period of the 1960s and 1970s, but became less effective during the 1980s. Because of the economic necessity of cutting back on budgets, the national government has in fact attempted to define and

Dena Shenk is Coordinator of the Gerontology Program and Professor of Anthropology at the University of North Carolina at Charlotte (UNCC). Kitter Christiansen lives in Løkken, Denmark, has a graduate degree in Psychology, and is a family counsellor. She completed early work at the Løkken-Vra research site as a part of her graduate work at Aalborg University Center.

Research completed in 1990 was funded by a St. Cloud (Minnesota) State University Research Grant and research completed in 1992 was funded by a UNCC Summer Research Grant to Dena Shenk.

[Haworth co-indexing entry note]: "The Evolution of the System of Care for the Aged in Denmark," Shenk, Dena, and Kitter Christiansen. Co-published simultaneously in the *Journal of Aging & Social Policy*, (The Haworth Press, Inc.) Vol. 5, No. 1/2, 1993, pp. 169-186; and: *International Perspectives on State and Family Support for the Elderly* (ed: Scott A. Bass and Robert Morris) The Haworth Press, Inc., 1993, pp. 169-186. Multiple copies of this article/chapter may be purchased from The Haworth Document Delivery Center [1-800-3-HAWORTH; 9:00 a.m. - 5:00 p.m. (EST)].

169

redirect available choices in service delivery. The dual themes of consistency and dynamism are demonstrated through the case of a rural municipality in northwest Jutland during the prosperous period into the more economically limited period of the last decade and the present. Implications for informal social support and relationships between the aged and their families, friends, and neighbors in Denmark are explored.

Formal services for the elderly in Denmark are based on a strong and consistent philosophical tradition of comprehensive social welfare focused on meeting the basic rights of every individual.[1] A related Danish belief suggests that survival through hard times depends upon cooperation–not competition (Thomas, 1990, p. 45). In Denmark, formal services are viewed as a *right* to be used by any member of that society who is in need of assistance, premised upon a societal model of mutual self-help.

Within this traditional framework, the Danish social welfare and health service delivery system is dynamic and seemingly in constant transition. Based on the social policy of viewing each individual as independent, a policy that was strongly supported during the economic boom of the 1960s and 1970s, the elderly came to regard formal services and not their family or friends as the appropriate way to meet their basic needs. The elderly Danish women in our study are reluctant to "lean" on family and friends when they are in need of basic help, expecting these needs to be met by formal service providers.[2] In the 1980s, however, the system tried to shape the demands of the elderly based on the limitations created by economic constraints.

The dual themes of philosophical consistency and change will be demonstrated in the case of a rural municipality in northern Denmark. The case of Løkken-Vra exemplifies a formal system of care for older adults with a firm philosophical base, which, however, has been refined continually and adjusted, first, to better meet the basic needs of the elderly, but more recently to accommodate the economic constraints of the 1980s.

Denmark is a country with 5.1 million people and 15.5% of the population are 65 or older. Denmark has a strong tradition of decentralized government with 15 counties (*amter*) and 275 municipalities (*kommuner*). Policy for medical and social services is set at the national level, but the actual operation of programs is at the level of municipalities and counties. Typically, new initiatives have been developed at the municipal level and then spread through legislation by the Parliament (Friis, 1979, p. 201). This process of creative development at the local level within the framework of policy set at the national level is demonstrated through the Løkken-Vra case study.

The system of formal services and programs to meet the basic needs of older adults is one component of the larger Danish system that provides for the basic needs of all citizens. The system of health and welfare services is financed essentially by the income taxes paid by all workers which begin at 51% of earned income. Services are free of charge for all residents, except for certain services provided by nursing homes and social welfare. For these services there are sliding fee scales for those earning more than a basic pension.

The responsibility of providing for the basic needs of all citizens is shared between the county and municipal levels of government with the national government providing partial reimbursement in the form of lump sum subsidies. Ownership of hospitals and provision of hospital and medical care services is at the county level.[3] The municipalities are responsible for the range of formal services necessary to meet the needs of elderly in their community. These services include nursing homes, day nursing homes, home nursing services, home help, meals-on-wheels, day centers, and sheltered housing.

The social welfare system in Denmark is based on the concepts of normalization and equalization. The concept of normalization has been described in regard to the mentally retarded as providing the same opportunities and conditions of life to the handicapped as are available to the rest of society and the right to experience and use the environment in a normal way (Bednar, 1976, p. 13). According to John McRae (1975, p. 28), "For many years, the primary goal of Danish social policies has been social equalization, where few have too much but fewer have too little." High priority is placed on providing services that preserve and strengthen the capabilities of the dependent elderly, particularly on services that will enable them to remain in their homes as long as possible (Raffel & Raffel, 1987). The basic orientation of the system of service delivery is toward maintaining the elderly's control over choices and enabling them to lead their lives as independently as possible.

While Denmark developed a comprehensive system of high-quality, government-financed services during the economically strong period prior to 1980, the government is struggling in this new economic climate. Officials are trying to maintain the level of services in spite of budget reductions, increased numbers of older adults, and increased demand for expensive medical technology (Raffel & Raffel, 1987). The case study demonstrates the evolution of the formal system struggling to meet the basic needs of the elderly in culturally acceptable ways in light of recent economic demands.

HISTORICAL BACKGROUND

Several historical developments are key to an understanding of Danish social policy for health and social welfare services for the elderly. These developments shaped the basic framework with which these elderly Danes have lived throughout their lives and form the basis for their expectations. The democratic constitution, which was introduced in 1849, guaranteed assistance to every citizen toward meeting his or her needs. From this early point, assistance was viewed by Danes as a legal right and substance was first given to this "right" with the passage of the Old Age Assistance Act in 1891. When the separate Acts of social legislation were combined in 1933, a comprehensive policy was formulated.

The next major changes took place during the booming economic era of the 1960s and 1970s. By the mid-1960s, the system of services was confusing and difficult to understand and the social reform of the 1970s focused on both improving and unifying the regulations (Fejerskov, 1989, p. 5). Passed in 1974, the Social Assistance Act included the introduction of the principle of treating the individual as a whole person, rather than a series of needs. It also included the beginning of the "one-stringed system" which required that an individual make application to a single local government office when in need of assistance.

Intensive debate on the conditions of the elderly was renewed in

1978, and called for a re-examination of the system with a focus on the needs and expectations of the elderly themselves. The National Commission on Aging established in 1979 produced three reports, including recommendations for improving old-age policy. As the 1980s began, however, the Danes saw the beginning of a changing economic reality, which no longer allowed continual expansion of formal services and unlimited spending.

Important changes were implemented with the 1984 Pension Reform and in 1987 with the "senior citizens' package." This package was the first serious attempt to formulate a comprehensive old-age policy, and treated the economic, physical, and social needs of the elderly in "light of the basic principles of self-determination, continuity, and the use of their own resources" (Fejerskov, 1989, p. 10). One objective of this plan was the "opening up" of nursing homes to the people of the neighborhood so they could participate in the activities.

Since the reforms of the 1970s, the emphasis has been on community-based care, which enables elders to remain in their own homes rather than moving to an institutional setting. There is a commitment to offer the same services to elders remaining in their own homes as those offered to nursing home residents. These changes are based on the concepts of normalization and equalization. The ability of the Danes to meet effectively the basic needs of the elderly has also been tempered by the changing economic realities and need to cut spending.

During the boom years, home health care (home-help) and home nursing services were utilized extensively in all of the Scandinavian countries of Denmark, Finland, Iceland, Norway, and Sweden. By the early 1980s, Denmark had both the highest volume and intensity of home help service among the Scandinavian countries (Daatland, 1986, p. 13). In Denmark not only were more clients being served but there was both a broadening and deepening of services, including night and weekend assistance (Daatland, 1986, p. 14). The economic constraints of the 1980s led to cutbacks in the availability of these home-based services.

The availability of formal services for the elderly in Denmark has changed since the 1970s along with the economic changes. During the 1970s, the situation was characterized by the motto "ask and you will receive," and elders received home help daily. During the 1980s, there was a need for recognition of the fact that services could not be expanded continually. Officials undertook an assessment of what the elderly really needed and attempted to move from "help" to "self-help." In the 1990s, there is a strong effort to help elders remain in their own homes as long as possible, in control of decisions about their environment (normalization) and as independent as possible, but the formal services that they have come to expect to support them in these efforts are no longer readily available.

Each municipality is required to establish a home help service and to provide free home nursing service upon referral from the patients' doctor. The type of home help that is particularly pertinent to the aged is permanent home help. It assists with domestic work that cannot be performed by a person with a permanent handicap or who is in frail health or permanently impaired. The work of the home helpers consists of part-time assistance with cleaning, washing, shopping, personal hygiene, dressing, and similar services. Actual nursing is done by the home nurse service. Some municipalities have or are planning to have coordination of the work of the home nurses and home helpers by a joint executive in charge of both services or through home care centers (Friis, 1979, p. 204-205). We will see herein how this system has developed in the case of the Løkken-Vra community.

The focus on remaining in control of one's own life is now being used to urge elders to care for themselves and each other. The recent development of formal services for the aged in Denmark has centered around the theme of "self-help" and has been forwarded through the development of experimental projects. While these efforts are necessitated by the economic strains that are currently being experienced in Denmark, they are also part of the effort to find positive and creative alternatives that can enable the elderly to remain active and independent. The Fynsgade Center in Aalborg, in the same county as Løkken-Vra, has become a model of a multi-service center that also includes sheltered housing. The community center Koltgarden in Arhus is another example of a center that "contains activities aimed at promoting good health, preventing disease and stimulating cultural endeavors" (Wolleson, 1989, p.

19). These are other examples of the country-wide efforts to "open up" nursing homes and move towards "self-help" in providing for the basic needs of the elderly in Denmark.

The social and health welfare system for the aged in Denmark is recognized as an advanced system. The Danes, however, continue to focus on problems and limitations in the system, working to improve the formal service delivery system within the constraints of the current economic situation. Their goals are as consistent as the constant transition that is evident in this dynamic system. The formal system of service delivery is designed to enable all individuals to live as normal a life as possible, assisted by their choice of services to meet their basic needs.

CASE STUDY OF LØKKEN-VRA

The Løkken-Vra municipality on the northwest coast of Jutland is a small municipality in the far corner of what was formerly referred to as "dark Jutland." Løkken and Vra were two separate municipalities that were combined in 1970[4] and comprise a population of 8,962. In this small rural municipality, we see dedicated attention to meeting the on-going needs of the elderly in creative and innovative ways. The dynamism in this system of formal service delivery for the elderly is built upon the consistent base of beliefs that has already been described. All individuals retain the right to have their basic needs met by a system of formal services that allows them to remain in control of their choices and their lives.

The area includes the towns of Løkken, Vrensted, and Vittrup. Løkken, now a seaside resort, was initially a seaport and later one of Denmark's larger fishing towns. Vrensted was a larger center and Vittrup a smaller center for the surrounding farming areas. They are both currently merely clusters of houses and farms surrounded by open country. A few stores including a grocery are all that remain of each community.

The inhabitants of the area are known as tough and independent people and were predominantly small farmers and fishermen.[5] The Borglum Monastery (Kloster) was active in the community from about 1130 until the 16th century and employed many local people.

Then, as a lay manor house, it continued to have a great impact on life in the area until the present. Because of technological advances, it is now run by a few people. A railway line went through the area, but the former Hjorring-Løkken-Aabybro railway was closed in 1963. The former station houses in Vrensted and Vittrup are now private residences.

The Løkken Museum was established in an old coastal fishing captain's house in the center of Løkken in 1978. The museum is notable because the restoration of the house and much of the work was done by volunteers. The museum works for preservation of the old Løkken environment, especially as it pertained to fishing. As we will see, this strong community spirit has also had an impact on the center for the aged.

There have been several notable steps in the process of integrating the formal service delivery system for the aged in Løkken-Vra. A director (*leder*) was hired in 1986 to arrange the closing of the old nursing home in Løkken and develop the new facility in Løkken, designed as a center of aging services. As outlined in the original job description, the responsibilities of the Director of the Elder Center (*centerleder*) included coordination of the multiple functions of the center and cooperation with the community and the other organizations that are important to the daily functioning of the center.

The original plans were outlined in a "Declaration of the Objectives for the Elder Center in Løkken" in 1986, the year before the implementation of the senior citizen's package nationally. As stated in the declaration, the elder center was intended to function as an open institution and an integral part of the local community and enable as many individuals as possible to stay in their own homes for as long as possible if that was what they wanted. Although these plans were developed a year in advance of the national senior citizen's package, they incorporated several aspects of that national plan. Part of the national attempt to formulate a comprehensive national old-age policy was the objective of "opening up" nursing homes to the people of the neighborhood so that they could participate. This goal was stated as well in the *Declaration of the Objectives for the Elder Center in Løkken*. The focus of the comprehensive old-age policy was to view the economic, physical, and social

needs of the elderly in terms of the basic principles of self-determination, continuity, and the use of their own resources. These
goals are clearly reflected as well in the Løkken document.

The *Declaration of the Objectives* gave creativity and experimental thinking a high priority in creating the center, as it stressed
the importance of an open atmosphere and availability of information for the pensioners. Residents and participants were to be
assisted in staying active and making their own decisions regarding
daily life. The center was also to be "adaptable to changing needs
and demands within the framework determined by legislation and
the local authorities" (*Declaration of the Objectives for the Elder
Center in Løkken*, n.d.).

Havgarden, as the center was named, includes a nursing home,
protected housing, a day center, and an open day center. There are
22 nursing home beds and 12 protected housing units. There are
four beds for "relief, training, and visiting" and four additional
temporary nursing home beds. These are used by people in transition between the hospital and home. There is a central kitchen and
the central watch for the 24-hour home care system. A day center
operates every weekday for participants who have been referred
because of their needs for daytime care. An open day center is
available to anyone in the community on Tuesday afternoons. The
participants play cards and do crafts.

Coordination of services is an essential element to a comprehensive plan that attempts to meet the individual's basic needs. In the
original *Declaration of Objectives,* the relationship of the Director
of the Elder Center with the Department of Home Health Care was
specifically clarified. A section concerning the administration of the
system of home health aides for the residents of the protected housing units of the center identified the Director as the contact person
for the Department of Home Health Care, which is responsible for
the visitation and for the staff who are working as home health
aides.

Significantly, Havgarden has been used and viewed as an essential community center for the surrounding community. Various
groups use the meeting rooms for planning meetings and community activities. For example, an event was held in June 1992 to
incorporate the newly arrived Kurdish population. The Kurds

cooked for the 90 people who attended the event and used the kitchen at Havgarden. A local cultural group called Løkken-Suset meets there regularly and holds activities including bimonthly dinners. Community residents as well as residents of Havgarden participate in these events. Havgarden is viewed as an integral component of the community and a community resource. Members of the community come and go freely, stopping by for a cup of coffee and to visit with staff and residents.

Most of the key staff have worked at Havgarden since the facility was opened in 1986. A notable exception is the Elder Leader, who was recently hired when the Director of the Elder Center resigned to take a new position. During the interim, while the position was being redefined and interviews were being conducted, community members filled the void. Collective management was instituted and volunteers worked with the Acting Director to continue social activities and community involvement in the Elder Center. Havgarden has "opened up" to this extent and community members clearly feel a responsibility for those who are living there. The efforts to meet the basic needs of the residents of Havgarden during the redefinition of the position remained within the framework of formal rather than informal supports.

The Elected Council of Løkken-Vra took this opportunity to implement a major change, reportedly in an effort towards further integration of the system of care for the aged in the municipality. The office of the home helpers has been relocated at Havgarden, apparently an effort to share resources and necessitated by the current economic decline. As stated in the advertisement for the current Director's position, "in connection with this decision, important changes will take place in the very near future in order to make the spending of resources in this field correspond to an offering of a greater diversification of services for the aged in the municipality." The move is towards a highly integrated system of services for the elderly in the municipality, headed by the Elder Leader. This change reflects the goals and guidelines we have discussed at the national level. In particular, providing a broader range of service options allows individuals to make choices that are more likely to meet their personal needs and enable them to control their environment. A well-integrated system of services is more likely to meet the needs of the whole individual and, again, enable the individual to live as normally as possible. Although not stated, it seems clear that a well-integrated system can also offer more services to more older individuals with less in funds.

The new position has changed dramatically from the original position of Director of the Elder Center. The new Elder Leader is responsible for the integrated system of care for the aged in regard both to professional nursing and administration. The Elder Leader is meant to play a central role in the process of change, and therefore has a great opportunity to participate in the creation both of the future structure and her own position.

The new Elder Leader began her job in May 1992. In an interview, she shared her understanding that her new position includes many parts; she is not just the Director of Havgarden (Marie, 1992). She is in charge of the 24-hour nursing program, home help, and Havgarden. It is a complex position which requires the juggling of priorities and satisfying many people. It is also a cost-saving measure, since her job now includes more components than the original leader's position.

Local leaders, including the Social Inspector and the Director of the Elder Center, designed and planned a Collective Health Project (*Kollectiv Sundhed*) for the Løkken-Vra municipality under a grant from a national social development fund created by the National Health Department. They hired a project director and completed the planning in August 1989. Unfortunately, when they applied for money from the National Health Department to implement the plan, they received no further funding because the fund had run short of money.

In 1990, there was a reduction in the number of hospitals throughout Denmark as a cost-saving measure. The Geriatric Hospital in Aalborg, in the same county as Løkken-Vra, was one of the hospitals closed. Parallel to the reduction in the number of hospitals, administrative officials in the county decided to work for the furthering of health and prevention of disease. These efforts were again driven by the economic constraints being felt throughout Denmark. A survey was completed in the 27 municipalities throughout the county of North Jutland (*Nordjyllands Amt*). Health Center Agreements were offered to the municipalities by officials of the county based on the

Health Profile (*Sundhedsprofil*) completed in each municipality. Sixteen municipalities were interested in the Health Center Agreements and four were chosen by the county officials. As one of these four communities, Løkken-Vra is scheduled to hire a new Health Center Coordinator.

As these two approaches to the improvement of health care and services for the elderly are based on similar ideas, grassroots and administrative planning have developed hand-in-hand. Both the Collective Health Project of Løkken-Vra and the official health policy that shapes the health program of the county (*Nordjyllands Amts Sundhedsplan*) are based on the Alma Ata Declaration about primary health care from the World Health Organization/UNICEF Conference of 1978.

Collaboration by the staff at Havgarden and citizens representing local community groups based on Project Collective Health reflects the view of care for the elderly in this community (Petersen & Christiansen, 1992). These community groups jointly presented a proposal to the chairman of the Løkken-Vra Social Committee and the Social Inspector concerning the formulation of future policy for the aged in the municipality. The Havgarden staff and local citizens suggested that Havgarden might be in the process of becoming a center of "culture" more than just a center for the aged. In the proposal they state: "to us this process is very fascinating and it might be a good idea to view it in connection to the Project Collective Health (*Kollektiv Sundhed*) and the *Sundhedsprofil* (Health Profile) of Løkken-Vra municipality." They point to "trends in social and health care policy which are blowing in the direction of the strengthening of local and volunteering powers, in the direction of growing responsibility of the citizens–to mention just a couple of ideas that have substance when you talk about Havgarden" (Petersen & Christiansen, 1992). The recommendations of the proposal include a thorough analysis of the well-being of the residents, the staff members, and other users of Havgarden as well as reconsideration and reformulation of the original objectives. The proposal's authors also recommend that a Health Board (*Sundhedsrad*) be established in accordance with the model described in Project Collective Health. These efforts are in accord with the national goals of normalization and equalization, and efforts to create a better-integrated system of formal care. They also reflect current efforts to increase the responsibility of local citizens in caring for the elderly, although still within the formal rather than the informal sector.

The proposal begins to identify how the recommendations of Project Collective Health can be implemented beginning with what is already occurring at Havgarden. It underlines the fact that the history of Havgarden runs parallel to the intentions of the Health Center agreements.

County officials are using the recently published report of Løkken-Vra's health profile as the basis for the Health Center Agreement (*"Sadan star det til med din sundhed-og sundheden i din kommune!" Sundhedsprofil for Løkken-Vra*, 1992). Negotiations are currently under way regarding which issues will be studied further. High priority will be given to the elderly's experience with stress. The health profile of Løkken-Vra shows that 23% of the oldest citizens indicated that they "most often" have a feeling of stress in daily life. Based on this finding, a proposal has been presented for a project entitled "The Aged and Stress," which would target the population of 513 citizens aged 80 years and older in Løkken-Vra. Research would focus on the causes of and avoidance of stress and how health promotion, disease prevention, and rehabilitation can be used to create effective health care services for the aged in the future. The program will be designed and carried out as a joint project between the Health Center Coordinator, Elder Leader, and home care nurses.

So, it is again (or still) a time of change in the Løkken-Vra municipality in regard to serving the needs of the aged through formal services. There is a new Elder Leader, holding a newly expanded and reformulated position, through which the municipality hopes to do more with less funding. A new Health Center Project is beginning that conforms to the design outlined in the local Collective Health Plan; it will certainly include specific projects focusing on the needs of the elderly. The local officials and community volunteers are creative in their search for new ways to offer comprehensive services to meet the basic needs of the elderly with the limited funds that are now available.

IMPLICATIONS FOR INFORMAL SOCIAL SUPPORT

The Danish view is that in order to get the necessary *social* support from family, friends, and neighbors, one must have to have one's basic needs met from somewhere else, that is, through formal services. The national government is encouraging a change in attitudes because of the economic necessity of cutting back on formal services. The elderly still receive formal services because "it is more acceptable. You can receive formal services without losing face" (Christiansen, 1992). The current effort is to get people to care more and to develop the informal system of care through which people help and support each other, as the economic situation worsens.

These views were expressed in response to a series of questions about both past and future use of formal services by the 30 older women in the Løkken-Vra study sample. While relatively few of the women had used each of these services, many of them indicated that they would use each of the services if they needed them in the future (see Table 1). In fact, one of the Danish informants got annoyed with these questions, indicating that the services are "a right."

The women were asked to whom they would turn for assistance

Table 1. Past and Future Use of Formal Services

	Denmark
Have used legal services	1
Would use legal services	28
Have used home-delivered meals	3
Would use home-delivered meals	28
Have used house-cleaning	9
Would use house-cleaning	27
Have used home-helper	13
Would use home-helper	28

with different needs and tasks. While there were variations in the numbers based on the kind of assistance needed, similar patterns were found. For help with paperwork or if they needed money, for example, the Danish women turned to professionals for help and less often to children, neighbors, and friends. In personal communications, informants also indicated that they would feel uncomfortable asking for help from friends or family.

The Danish system of services can be explained in terms of the cultural value of privacy. When money was available, formal services were used more because of this pattern of maintaining privacy. Those in need wanted to stay protected and private and would turn to formal services rather than ask friends or even family for help.

Older Danish women are comfortable accepting formal services, but not necessarily asking friends and family for assistance. The elderly are willing to use formal services because, as we have already discussed, that is viewed as acceptable and a "right," and one can receive these services without losing face. It is not always easy, however, for elders to request the assistance they need from friends or even family. The current effort at the national level in Denmark is to get people in the informal sector to "care" more, to develop the informal system of care through which people help and support each other, as the economic situation worsens. Clearly, each society must develop a framework for effective interaction of the formal and informal systems of care in meeting the basic physical and social needs of the elderly that is based on cultural expectations (see Shenk, 1992).

CONCLUSIONS

Formal services are viewed as a *right* to be used by any member of Danish society who is in need of assistance, premised upon mutual self-help. Having one's basic needs met by formal services allows one to interact with friends and family on a more equal basis. Formal services are not viewed in Denmark as an approach to be used only when one's informal network is unable to meet one's needs. This fact is critical to our understanding of the system of informal and formal services for the elderly in Denmark. The Danish system of services appears to be a response to the societal preference for using formal services to meet basic needs, allowing the individual to depend on informal supports to meet social needs. The system now clearly perpetuates that preference. In order to keep up the high level of the formal support system during a period of economic regression, more efficient utilization of the available funds will depend on several factors. The focus should be on strengthening the independence of the individual, introduction of a policy of prevention, involvement of each citizen on all levels in these efforts, and the sharing of responsibility. Responsibility for meeting the basic needs of the elderly cannot merely be redirected from the formal support system to the informal system of support without regard for cultural expectations.

The case study of Løkken-Vra has been presented to demonstrate the dynamic nature of the system of care for elders in Denmark and the example of a small rural county as a progressive place for experiments in the field of services for the elderly. At the same time it exemplifies the consistency provided by the clear philosophical belief in the rights of each individual to receive appropriate care. In order to maintain high standards and continue to develop a society that develops autonomy throughout the lifecycle, the Danes must continue to create new ways to improve their quality of life. The adaptation of the new health policy in Løkken-Vra might be one of these new ways. Within this context, the developments in small, local communities like Løkken-Vra take on great significance. It might very well be that the next step in a society like Denmark is to develop models for the formal social service system that are based on true equality between all of the players—professionals as well as consumers. And it might be that this process of creation demands personal contact between the individuals through the personal confrontation that can only take place in local society, where they know each other personally.

While there are clearly limitations on the policy implications we can draw from this case of a rural municipality in the tiny country of Denmark, we believe there are valuable lessons to be learned from this example. This case demonstrates the advantage of building a service delivery system on a firm and consistent philosophical base, which provides the basis for shared expectations among members of the society. This consistency also allows for the development of the second strength that we have identified in the Danish system of service delivery. The Danish example demonstrates the effectiveness of a dynamic system of service delivery, which responds to changing and developing needs, rather than a static, inflexible system. Unfortunately, the current changes are apparently controlled by economic necessity as well as the loftier goals of normalization and equalization. The Danish system also demonstrates the possibilities of allowing individuals to retain control over their own lives and choices for alternative ways of meeting their needs.

NOTES

1. This philosophical tradition is exemplified by the work of Soren Kierkegaard, the Danish philosopher, who stated: "If real success is to attend the effort to bring a man to a definite position, one must first of all take pains to find HIM where he is and begin there. This is the secret of the art of helping others. Anyone who has not mastered this is himself deluded when he proposes to help others. In order to help another effectively I must understand more than he–yet first of all surely I must understand what he understands. If I do not know that, my greater understanding will be of no help to him" (Bretall, 1951).

2. The research on which this discussion is based was completed in Løkken-Vra on the northwest coast of North Jutland, Denmark. The case study is based on participant observation and questionnaire data from a sample of 30 older women in Løkken-Vra. The sample was selected during the summer of 1990, based on earlier work by the second author. The interviews were conducted by the second author in the summer and fall of 1990, and the first author completed a follow-up visit in May 1992.

3. In an effort to adjust to the current economic problems, a system of private medical care is developing as an alternative for those willing to pay for medical services.

4. On April 1, 1970, the number of municipalities was cut from nearly 1,000 to 278 and the number of counties from 22 to 14, plus the two municipalities of Copenhagen and Frederiksberg (geographically part of Copenhagen), which have status as counties.

5. An ethnographic culture study by Anderson and Anderson, 1964 (see also Anderson, 1990) provides a picture of life in a similar fishing community outside of Copenhagen at the turn of the 19th and 20th centuries.

REFERENCES

Anderson, R.T., & Anderson, B.G. (1964). *The vanishing village: A Danish maritime community.* Seattle: University of Washington Press.

Anderson, B.G. (1990). *First fieldwork: The misadventures of an anthropologist.* Prospect Heights, Illinois: Waveland Press.

Bednar, M. (1974). *Architecture for the handicapped: Denmark, Sweden and Holland.* Ann Arbor: The University of Michigan.

Bretall, R. (1951). *A Kierkegaard Anthology.* Translation of S. Kierkegaard, *The point of view for my work as an author,* Part 2, chapter 1, section 2.3333. Princeton, NJ: Princeton University Press.

Christiansen, K. (1992, May 19). Personal communication.

Daatland, S. O. (1986, Spring). Nordic countries emphasize community care. *Aging International, 13* (1), 13-14.

Declaration of the Objectives for the Senior Center in Løkken. No date. Unpublished document.

Fejerskov, R. (1989). Danish old-age policy. In *The elderly in Denmark* (pp. 5-10). Copenhagen: The Danish Cultural Institute.

Friis, H. (1979). The aged in Denmark: Social programmes. In M.I. Teicher, D. Thursz, and J. Vigilante (Eds.), *Reaching the aged: Social services in forty-four countries* (pp. 201-211). Beverly Hills: Sage Publications.

Marie, A. (1992, May 19). Personal communication.

McRae, J. (1975). *Elderly in the environment: Northern Europe.* Gainesville, Florida: College of Architecture and Center for Gerontological Studies and Programs.

Petersen, G., & Christiansen, K. (1992). *Concerning the formulation of the future policy of the aged in our municipality.* Unpublished manuscript.

Peterson, J. (1990, January). The Danish 1891 Act on Old Age Relief: A response to agrarian demand and pressure. *Journal of Social Policy, 19,* 69-91.

Raffel, N., & Raffel, M. (1987, September-October). Elderly care: Similarities and solutions in Denmark and the United States. *Public Health Reports, 102,* 494-500.

"Sadan star det til med din sundhed–og sundheden i din kommune!" Sundhedsprofil for Løkken-Vra Kommune ("This is the state of your health–and the health in your municipality!") Health Profile of Løkken-Vra Municipality (1992). Nordjyllands Amt (County of North Jutland), Denmark.

Shenk, D. (1992, December). *Support systems of rural older women in Denmark and Minnesota.* Paper presented at the meeting of the American Anthropological Association, San Francisco.

Shenk, D. (1991). Older rural women as recipients and providers of social support. *Journal of Aging Studies, 5*(4), 347-358.

Shenk, D. (1987). *Someone to lend a helping hand: The lives of rural older women in Central Minnesota.* St. Cloud: Central Minnesota Council on Aging.

Teicher, M.I., Thursz, D., & Vigilante, J. (Eds.) (1979). *Reaching the aged: Social services in forty-four countries.* Beverly Hills: Sage Publications.

Thomas, F. R. (1990). *Americans in Denmark: Comparisons of the two cultures by writers, artists and teachers.* Carbondale: Southern Illinois Press.

Wolleson, A.M. (1989). Koltgarden: From idea to reality. In L. Lichtenberg and K. Hegelund (Eds.), *The elderly in Denmark* (pp.19-22). Copenhagen: The Danish Cultural Institute.

Understanding the Pattern of Support for the Elderly: A Comparison Between Israel and Sweden

Jack Habib, PhD

JDC-Brookdale Institute of Gerontology
and Human Development, Jerusalem

Gerdt Sundstrom, PhD

Institute of Gerontology, Jonkoping, Sweden

Karen Windmiller, MPH

Lincoln Gerontology Centre
Melbourne, Australia

SUMMARY. Cross-cultural comparison can offer critical input to analyses of the interplay between formal and informal services for

Jack Habib is Senior Researcher at the JDC-Brookdale Institute of Gerontology and Human Development in Israel and Associate Professor in the Departments of Economics and Social Work at the Hebrew University in Jerusalem. Gerdt Sundstrom is Associate Professor at the University of Stockholm and is Senior Researcher at the Institute of Gerontology at Jonkoping, Sweden. Karen Windmiller is a Research Fellow at the Lincoln Gerontology Centre at La Trobe University (Abbotsford campus) in Melbourne, Australia.

This article is based on a paper presented to the XIV Congress of the International Association of Gerontology in Acapulco, Mexico in June 1989.

[Haworth co-indexing entry note]: "Understanding the Pattern of Support for the Elderly: A Comparison Between Israel and Sweden," Habib, Jack, Gerdt Sundstrom, and Karen Windmiller. Co-published simultaneously in the *Journal of Aging & Social Policy,* (The Haworth Press, Inc.) Vol. 5, No. 1/2, 1993, pp. 187-206; and: *International Perspectives on State and Family Support for the Elderly* (ed: Scott A. Bass and Robert Morris) The Haworth Press, Inc., 1993, pp. 187-206. Multiple copies of this article/chapter may be purchased from The Haworth Document Delivery Center [1-800-3-HAWORTH; 9:00 a.m. - 5:00 p.m. (EST)].

© 1993 by The Haworth Press, Inc. All rights reserved.
187

the elderly. Israel and Sweden have very different population structures and represent different points on the spectrum of welfare state development: Sweden has a much higher percentage of elderly, a less traditional family structure, and a much more developed system of public support. In addition, there are thought to be different attitudes toward family ties, with a less family-oriented value structure in Sweden. The natural question is to what extent these differences translate into differences in the extent and nature of family support for the elderly.

In this article, family structure, living arrangements, disability rates, and formal and informal sources of help in Sweden and Israel are compared at various points in time. While there is a greater rate of formal service provision in Sweden and some substitution for family support seems to have occurred, informal care has nevertheless remained important. In both countries, residential patterns are critical: it is when the elderly live alone that the formal system has tended to replace the family. The rate of institutionalization is particularly important in determining the rate of disabled elderly requiring care, both formal and informal, in the community.

The roles of formal and informal support in the care of the elderly have been a major focus of concern and research among policymakers. A central issue has been the degree to which the development and expansion of formal services leads to a reduction in informal support. Surprisingly, evaluations of new programs in the United States have found little evidence of substitution; formal services tend to supplement existing informal services rather than replace them. (For a summary of this research, see Habib & Cohen, 1990 and Kemper, Applebaum, & Harrigan, 1990.) It has been suggested that the provision of formal services may cause family members to shift their efforts to other types of aid (Greene, 1983, and Lewis, Binstock, Cantor, & Schneewind, 1980), but these findings have not been replicated by experimental demonstration project evaluations.

The San Diego Long Term Care Program (Pinkerton & Hill, 1984) and the national Financial Model Channeling Demonstration (Christianson, 1988), both conducted in the United States, found no decrease in help with ADL (activities of daily living) tasks. They reported some decrease in informal help with IADL (instrumental activities in daily living) tasks, but in the Channeling evaluation the effects were only statistically significant at the six-month follow-up and subsequently disappeared. Moreover, where help was withdrawn, it seems to have occurred mainly among those least closely associated with the client, namely, friends and neighbors and relatives other than spouses or children who do not live with the elderly person. The total number of visits per week and total number of hours of care from all informal caregivers were not affected by formal support services, nor was the amount of help from the primary caregiver (Christianson, 1988).

Another source of input on this critical issue is the analysis of cross-country variations. Has the informal system been replaced or significantly reduced in societies with changing age and social structures and older, more advanced welfare states? Has the change been universal or focused on certain population subgroups or situations? The Scandinavian countries have well-established welfare states, and there have been conflicting claims with respect to the present status of informal support in these societies. On the one hand, it has been argued that the family is no longer a major provider of personal care and homemaking services (Andersson, 1985). Moreover, it has been suggested that the elderly do not want their children to provide these kinds of care but prefer public sources of provision (Daatland, 1990). In contrast, Henning Friis (1977) argues that studies in Denmark show that the introduction of services has not been accompanied by decreasing contact with or assistance to elderly parents on the part of adult children. Gerdt Sundstrom (1986) and Lars Tornstam (1989) contend that the informal support system is still very important, and that contact between old people and their children is more frequent than earlier believed.

In this article, we attempt to shed light on these roles by comparing two societies, Israel and Sweden, that have very different population structures and represent different points on the spectrum of welfare state development. We examine how basic societal structural differences such as family networks and living arrangements interact with dependency (i.e., requiring assistance in areas of personal care and in homemaking) among the elderly to affect care patterns. We also discuss the extent to which the different rates of formal support are accompanied by significant differences in informal support patterns. We emphasize an integrated perspective, with comparisons of total populations of elderly over the age of 65, including those living in the community as well as in institutions. Data on support to the elderly in Sweden in 1954 will also be presented to enable comparison of support patterns in the two societies at times when their demographic structures and the extent of public support were similar.

POPULATION DIFFERENCES
AND FORMAL SERVICE DEVELOPMENT

Israel and Sweden have very different age distributions. In 1985, 9.7% of the population in Israel was aged 65 and older, 4.5% aged 75 and over, and 2.1% aged 85 and over. In Sweden, the respective rates were significantly higher: 16.9% were 65 and older, 7.2% were 75 and older, and 3.5% were 85 and older. The ratio of elderly to the working age population was correspondingly much lower in Israel, 17.7% compared to 29.4% in Sweden (Torrey, Kinsella, & Taeuber, 1987).

In addition to these large differences in the age structure, there are considerable differences in basic family patterns in the two countries. Marriage and birth rates are considerably higher in Israel than in Sweden and divorce rates are lower. Sweden is at the forefront of changes in traditional family norms with high percentages of nonmarried adults, one-parent families, and children born out of wedlock (often born to parents who are not legally married but who live together as couples). In 1984, 1% of children born in Israel were illegitimate compared to 44.6% in Sweden (United Nations Demographic Yearbook, 1986).

Another point of comparison is the pattern of labor force participation for women. In Israel in 1972, 34% of women aged 45 to 54 and 24% of women aged 55 to 64 participated in the work force; in 1984, the figures were 46% and 26%, respectively (Torrey et al., 1987). In Sweden in 1975, 75% of women aged 45 to 54 and 50% of women aged 55 to 64 participated in the work force; by 1985, the figures were 88% and 60%, respectively (Johnson & Scott, 1988).

Despite these differences in some of the basic characteristics of the two societies, life expectancy is fairly similar. Life expectancy in Israel in 1985 was 73.9 years for men and 77.3 for women (Central Bureau of Statistics, 1987a); in Sweden in 1985, it was 73.8 years for men and 79.7 for women (United Nations Demographic Yearbook 1986). Sex differences in life expectancy are greater in Sweden, yet the overall ratio of males to females among the elderly is quite similar, with a difference emerging only among those aged 80 and older; there were a larger proportion of females in Sweden (64%) than in Israel (54%) (Torrey et al., 1987). Regarding the levels of services to the elderly, previous research has established the high rate of formal service provision in Sweden (Andersson, 1985; Daatland, 1985; Sundstrom, 1983, 1985, 1986) as well as the limited role of formal support in Israel (Habib, Factor, Naon, Brodsky, & Dolev, 1986; Morginstin, 1987; Morginstin & Werner, 1986).

SOURCES

This analysis was possible because of the availability of a survey in each country that integrates demographic data, data on needs, and data on helping patterns. For Sweden, this was the 1975 Survey of Elderly Persons (Statistics Sweden, 1977), which studied both institutionalized and noninstitutionalized elderly. The survey was conducted during the years when the provision of public services to the elderly was at its peak (G. Sundstrom, 1987). The national censuses, the Swedish Annual Level-of-Living Survey of 1980-1981, a study by Sundstrom (1984) about family networks, and the 1954 Swedish Survey of Elderly Persons (Statistics Sweden, 1956) were also most useful.

For Israel, we used the 1985 National Survey of the Elderly in the Community (Central Bureau of Statistics, 1988). Supplementary data on the institutionalized elderly were taken from a special survey conducted in 1981 (Factor, Guttman, & Shmueli, 1984). Other data were obtained from the national censuses and a number of special surveys, including a study on kinship networks (Shmueli, 1989).

THE NATURE OF THE INFORMAL SUPPORT NETWORK

In the 1980s, some 60% of the elderly in Israel were married as compared to 51% in Sweden. The percentage never married was much higher in Sweden (11 to 13%) than in Israel (2 to 3%). While a majority of the elderly in both societies have children, more than twice as many in Sweden are childless (23% in Sweden in 1980/81 versus 11% in Israel in 1985). These data suggest that informal support should be more available in Israel. The difference in the potential availability of informal support between Israel today and Sweden in 1954 is even greater because of the larger gap in marriage rates (see Table 1).

Overall, there is also quite a significant difference between the two countries in patterns of living arrangements. First of all, in Sweden in 1975 close to 7% of the elderly were living in institutions compared to 4% in Israel in 1985. Secondly, the percentage of older people living alone is very different in the two countries: 28% in Israel in 1985 and 38% in Sweden in 1986/87. This difference is for the most part explained by a difference in the rates of those living with children–18% in Israel in 1985, compared to 5% in Sweden in 1986/87.

A similar disparity is evident when we look at the percentage of elderly who are not married (i.e., never married, divorced, or widowed) and not living with children (subsequently referred to as the NMNLWC subgroup). This was 30% of all elderly in Israel in 1985 compared to 42% in Sweden in 1975 (Table 2). Over the years, the percentage living alone has increased in both societies and the percentage living with children has decreased.

A much larger percentage of Israeli elderly than Swedish elderly live with their children (Table 1)–18% in Israel (1985) versus 7% in Sweden (1980-81)–or in close proximity to them. In Israel, 41% live within 1.5 kilometers of at least one of their children, versus 33% in Sweden.

There are many forms of support for the elderly. It is important to distinguish between emotional support, which mainly relates to maintaining contact, and instrumental support, which relates to meeting daily personal care and homemaking needs. Some of the confusion in the literature with respect to the extent of family care and to trends over time is due to a failure to distinguish between these two types of support. In principle, formal services could provide both emotional and instrumental care; however, in practice, the formal care system tends to focus on instrumental care, with emotional support left to the informal care system.

If we briefly examine the evidence on emotional support as

TABLE 1. Marital Status and Household Structure for Elderly Aged 65 + in Israel and Sweden[2]

Marital Status[1]	Israel				Sweden				
	1961	1972	1983	1985	1954	1975	1976	1980-81	1987
Married	55	58	60	61	46	50	–	51	51
Widowed	40	38	35	35	37	31	–	31	31
Divorced	2	2	2	2	2	4	–	5	7
Never married	3	3	3	2	15	15	–	13	11
Total	100	100	100	100	100	100	–	100	100
Childless[2]	NA	NA	NA	11	23	NA	25	23	NA

Household structure[3]	Israel				Sweden			
	1961	1972	1983	1985	1954	1975	1980-81	1986-87
Alone	12	19	27	28	27	41	37	38
Spouse	35	45	51	52	33	46	52	54
Spouse & others[4]	21	15	10	10	11	5	4	3
Child	30	19	10	8	16	4	3	2
Other	2	2	2	2	13	4	4	3
Total[5]	100	100	100	100	100	100	100	100
% in Institutions	NA	NA	4	4	6	7	NA	NA

[1] Israel data for 1985 relate to noninstitutionalized elderly. The distribution of marital status and household structure is similar for aged 65+ and aged 65-84.
[2] Israel data refer to the noninstitutionalized. Sweden data refer to the total elderly.
[3] Israel data for 1961, 1972 and 1983 relate to Jews only.
[4] "Others" are almost exclusively children.
[5] Figures may not add up to 100% due to rounding.

SOURCES:

Israel: Central Bureau of Statistics, 1962, 1981, 1986, 1988; Be'er, S. and Factor, H. 1988; Noam, G. and Sicron, M. 1990.

Sweden: Sjoberg, I., 1990; Statistics Sweden, 1956, 1977, 1985a, 1985b; 1987.

TABLE 2. Living Arrangements and Dependency of the Elderly in Israel and Sweden (percentages)

	Living With Children		Not Living With Children				% of Total Pop. Aged 65+	Pop.² (thousands)
	Married¹	Not Married¹	Married¹	Not Married¹	Inst.	Total		
Total population aged 65+:								
Israel 1985	9	8	49	30	4	100	10	304.5
Sweden 1975	5	4	42	42	7	100	9	1081.0
Sweden 1954	10	15	31	38	6	100		638.0
Population aged 65 dependent in:								
Personal Hygiene:								
Israel 1985	9	20	26	21	24	100		30.0
Sweden 1975	5	4	9	12	70	100		102.4
Cleaning:								
Israel 1985	14	12	48	17	9	100	45	135.0
Sweden 1975	7	5	32	39	16	100	45	454.0
Shopping:								
Israel 1985	11	19	30	21	19	100	21	63.0
Sweden 1975	6	8	26	35	25	100	27	296.2
Sweden 1954	14	21	31	23	11	100	52	336.0
Cooking:								
Israel 1985	16	8	55	11	10	100	37	113.2
Sweden 1975	9	6	36	23	25	100	26	285.9
Mobility:³								
Israel 1985	10	18	33	26	13	100	18	53.8
Sweden 1975	2	5	19	44	30	100	12	158.0
Sweden 1954	8	16	24	32	19	100	20	127.6

[1] Not married refers to those never married, divorced, or widowed.
[2] Weighted figures.
[3] Outdoor mobility; can or cannot get around unaccompanied outdoors.

Sources   ISRAEL: Central Bureau of Statistics, 1988; Be'er, S. and Factor, H., 1988.

SWEDEN: Statistics Sweden, 1956, 1977.

reflected in frequency of contact, we find that although there is more contact between the elderly and their children in Israel, contact is also very extensive in Sweden. In 1985, 80% of Israeli elderly, including those who lived with children, saw their children at least once a week (Central Bureau of Statistics, 1988) compared to 68% of Swedish elderly in 1980-81 (Sundstrom, 1983). Only 13% of the elderly in Israel saw their children less than once a week but at least once a month, and 8% saw them seldom or not at all, compared with 19% and 13%, respectively, in Sweden.

DEPENDENCY, FAMILY STATUS, AND LIVING ARRANGEMENTS

Having identified some basic differences in potential informal support between Israel and Sweden, we now turn to an examination of the implications for the dependent elderly. We first present data on dependency rates and contrast the demographic status of the dependent and the independent. We have confined ourselves to a single data source for each country which has been manipulated so as to allow for maximum comparability.

Table 2 presents the dependency rates for the total elderly populations. Nine percent to 10% of the elderly in both countries are dependent on others for personal hygiene. However, the percentage dependent regarding mobility is considerably higher in Israel in 1985 (18%) than in Sweden in 1975 (12%).

One would expect a higher rate of dependency in Sweden because of the older age structure. However, there are apparently offsetting differences in the age-specific rates. This could be related to the higher levels of education and income, which are very highly correlated with dependency. There could also be a cultural difference in the tendency to perceive oneself as dependent or to report dependency.

The rates of dependency regarding homemaking vary considerably by type of activity and the gap between the two countries varies as well (see Table 2). In Sweden, the dependency rate is highest for cleaning (45%), while for shopping and cooking the rates are much lower and are similar (26% and 27%, respectively).

In Israel, the rate is also highest for cleaning (the same as that of Sweden—45%). Thirty-seven percent of the elderly in Israel are dependent on others for cooking and the rate is lowest for shopping (21%). Dependency regarding IADL, or daily living tasks, would appear to have a strong cultural component. It is related not only to what the individual is capable of doing, but also to what he or she has been culturally accustomed to doing. This latter factor is particularly influenced by sex roles. In Israel, there are gender-related norms for shopping and cooking. Men in Israel, particularly those of Middle Eastern origin, tend to assume the shopping role, whereas they would not generally take part in cooking. This may perhaps explain the much higher rate of dependency for cooking in Israel as compared to Sweden, and, by contrast, the lower rate for shopping. Sex differences are further explored in Habib, Sundstrom, and Windmiller (in press). Regardless of the source of these differences, they create differential needs for assistance.

We have seen in the previous section the major differences in the living arrangements of the elderly in Israel and Sweden, and the advantage of the Israeli elderly in terms of access to support. We now examine whether this carries over to the dependent elderly or whether there are compensating mechanisms at work. The difference in institutional rates among the overall population translates into a large difference in the institutional rates of those dependent regarding personal hygiene or mobility. Of those requiring help with personal hygiene, 70% live in institutions in Sweden, as compared with only 24% in Israel. Similarly, of those requiring help with mobility, 30% live in institutions in Sweden as compared with only 13% in Israel. For those dependent in IADL, the difference in the rates of institutionalization is much more limited.

The greater access to support of the Israeli elderly carries over to the dependent as well. Sweden has a higher percentage in the high-risk NMNLWC category for all dependent groups with the exception of those requiring personal care, of whom 70% are institutionalized. The difference in the rates of NMNLWC in Israel and Sweden is even greater for those with IADL limitations than it is for the elderly in general. At the same time, not surprisingly, the dependent elderly in both countries tend to live with their children more than do the independent elderly. However, because this tendency is greater in Israel, the gap between Israel and Sweden in the potential availability of informal support is wider. Living arrangements already reflect the differential involvement of informal sources of support. The elderly who live with their spouse or children most probably receive the range of services that are routinely provided to all members of the household. We examine actual support patterns in the next section.

THE ROLE OF FORMAL AND INFORMAL CARE

Considering the differences in potential informal support and living arrangements, we would expect informal support to play a much greater role in Israel than in Sweden. In this section, we analyze sources of support according to the following categories: spouse or other household member, family outside of household, friend or neighbor, help paid out-of-pocket, and public help.

While there may be more than one source of support for an elderly individual, the literature indicates that there is generally a primary supporter who provides most, if not all, of the needed care. In the 1975 Swedish Survey of Elderly Persons, dependent respondents were asked: "Who is your primary helper?" The Swedish survey did not include help paid out-of-pocket as a category, as it was not considered to be widely available. In the 1985 Israeli National Survey of Elderly in the Community and the 1954 Swedish Survey of Elderly Persons, respondents could cite more than one source of help.

In order to create a basis for comparison with the data from the 1975 Swedish survey, we assigned in our study persons in both the 1954 Swedish survey and the 1985 Israeli survey who were receiving support from more than one source a primary caregiver according to the following order: public help, spouse or other household member, family outside the household, friend or neighbor, help paid out-of-pocket. As the availability of public help was low, and as it was considered important to identify its full extent, it was given first priority. For example, if someone was receiving both public help and help from a household member, they were placed in the "public help" category. Similarly, persons who received help from both a household member and help paid out-of-pocket were placed in the "household member" category. The percentage of dependent elderly receiving help from more than one source was quite low. In Israel, it varied from 7% in the area of cleaning, to 5% in shopping, 2% in cooking, and 3% in personal hygiene. Moreover, approximately half of the persons who received help from more than one source were receiving help from both their spouse and another household member, which for the purpose of comparison with Sweden have been combined into the same category. Thus, we do not believe that this adjustment seriously limits the comparability of the data.

We found a very large difference in the percentage of dependent noninstitutionalized elderly receiving formal support in the two countries. In Israel, 8% of the dependent elderly population received formal support with hygiene, 7% with shopping, 3% with cleaning, and 2% with cooking. As a percentage of the total elderly, this represents 0.6%, 1%, 0.3%, 0.6%, respectively. In Sweden, by contrast, 25% of the dependent elderly population received formal support with personal hygiene, 44% with cleaning, 23% with shopping, and 16% with cooking. As a percentage of the total elderly, this represents 1%, 15%, 5%, and 3%, respectively. (Because of space limitations, only data on help with personal hygiene and shopping are presented–see Tables 3 and 4.)

Aside from the difference in total support between the two countries, there is a clear difference in emphasis. In Israel, relatively speaking, there is more of an emphasis on personal care, whereas in Sweden the emphasis is on homemaking.

Although there is a much higher rate of formal support in Sweden, it does not emerge as the primary source of support for either those with ADL or IADL limitations. This is true overall, and for the various subgroups, with one exception: those not married and not living with children. For the NMNLWC, public support predominates with respect to personal hygiene and cleaning (but not shopping or cooking). In both countries, formal support is concentrated on this subgroup.

For all other groups, most care is provided by the informal support system, with nonresident family members playing a significant part, especially in Israel. Resident family members, another impor-

TABLE 3. Source of Help for Noninstitutionalized Elderly Aged 65+ Requiring Help in Personal Hygiene (percentages)[1]

Total Population Dependent in Personal Hygiene[2]	Total	Living With Children or Married	Not Living With Children & Not Married
Israel (1985)			
Spouse/other household member	68	90	8
Family outside household	22	6	64
Friend/Neighbor	2	0	8
Public help	8	4	20
Total[3]	100	100	100
Pop. N (thousands)[4]	22.6	16.4	6.1
Percent dependent	8	8	7
Sweden (1975)			
Spouse/other household member	65	83	33
Family outside household	9	13	-
Friend/Neighbor	2	0	6
Public help	25	3	60
Total[3]	100		100
Pop. N (thousands)[4]	28.5	18.2	10.5
Percent dependent	3	3	2

[1] Missing values excluded (0.2% of total Swedish population; 0.8% of dependent Israel population). Israel category "no help" was excluded: (1% of respondents). Swedish category "not enough help" was excluded: (7% of respondents, all of whom are unmarried). Category "help paid out-of-pocket" not included in 1975 Swedish questionnaire.
[2] Dependent (Israel and Sweden): cannot manage without help of another person.
[3] Figures may not add up to 100 due to rounding.
[4] Weighted figures.

Sources   Israel: Central Bureau of Statistics, 1988.
               Sweden: Statistics Sweden, 1977.

TABLE 4. Source of Help for Noninstitutionalized (percentages)

Total Population Dependent in Shopping	Sweden, 1954	
	Total	NMNLWC
Source of Help		
Spouse/other household member	77	28
Family outside household	11	30
Friend/Neighbor/Other[2]	8	30
Help paid out-of-pocket[3]	3	8
Public help	1	4
Total[4]	100	100
Pop. N (thousands)[5]	294	76
Percentage dependent	49	32

[1] Dependent in shopping: Sweden 1954: do not do this activity themselves; Sweden 1975: cannot manage without help of another person; Israel 1985: have difficulty doing or cannot do this activity.
[2] In Sweden 1954, many of these persons lived with siblings, former employ- ers, ex-farmhands, lodgers, etc.
[3] No help paid out-of-pocket reported in Sweden in 1975.
[4] Figures may not add up to 100% due to rounding.
[5] Weighted figures.

tant source of informal care, are most often spouses in Sweden, while in Israel spouses and children are evenly represented.

Of particular interest are the differences in the informal support patterns for the NMNLWC group. In Israel, family outside the household dominate the care of the NMNLWC, while in Sweden support from family outside the household is virtually nonexistent for personal care in the NMNLWC group and relatively less fre- quent for the other areas of care. This may be due, in part, to the fact that, relative to Israel, in Sweden a higher percentage of NMNLWC receive care from other household members, usually siblings (co- residence with siblings is high among the never-married, who constitute a large group in Sweden), and from friends and neigh- bors.

In summary, the overall difference between Israel and Sweden in the role of public and family support is related to the difference in institutionalization rates, which particularly affects the provision of personal care needs; to the large difference in the degree of public support for one particular subgroup, the NMNLWC; and to the larger prevalence of this group among the Swedish dependent. However, contrary to expectations, the family continues to dominate the provision of care for homemaking needs in Sweden. In the case of personal care, public services predominate but only because of the high rate of institutionalization, which has been a long-term historical reality in Sweden. For elderly in the community, support by the family predominates, even for personal care. Again, in contrast to common perceptions, co-residence is the main vehicle of family support in both countries, with family outside the home playing a lesser role.

COMPARISON WITH SWEDEN IN 1954

In this section, we examine changes in Sweden over time and compare Israel in 1985 to Sweden in 1954, when the demographic structures and extent of public support in the two countries were quite similar. During the 1960s and 1970s, Sweden experienced dramatic changes in the age structure and a period of rapid growth of the welfare state. The percentage of elderly increased from 8.3% of Sweden's population in 1900 to 10.3% in 1951, and then leaped to 17.2% in 1985 (Johnson & Scott, 1988). In 1985, 8.9% of the Israeli population were aged 65 and over (Habib & Windmiller, 1992). The 1954 Swedish data also show a labor force participation rate among women similar to the current rate of women's labor force participation in Israel (Central Bureau of Statistics, 1987b; M. Sundstrom, 1987). The 1954 data also enable us to compare the two societies prior to the major expansion of the welfare state in Sweden, when the rates of provision of formal services were more similar than they are today.

In Sweden in 1954, many more elderly lived with children than in Israel in 1985 (16% in Sweden compared with 8% in Israel) but fewer lived with a spouse (33% compared with 52%–see Table 1). The difference in marital status patterns between Israel in 1985 and Sweden in 1954 reflects the impact of different social norms for given age structures. Countries today reaching the degree of aging that characterized Sweden in 1954 may have a very different pattern of living arrangements, particularly with respect to older people living with their children. This highlights the important interaction between the process of population aging and the change in living standards and norms.

Formal support was higher in Sweden both in 1954 and 1975 than in Israel in 1985 (see Table 4 for an analysis of sources of help in the area of shopping, as an example). The difference between Israel in 1985 and Sweden in 1954 is due to the higher rates of institutionalization in Sweden. These rates were relatively high in Sweden well before the major period of rapid aging and the development of the welfare state. The difference between Israel in 1985 and Sweden in 1975 is also due to the much higher rates of formal community services for elderly living in the community in Sweden at that time.

The analysis of Sweden over time and the comparison between Israel today and Sweden in earlier periods highlight the fact that support from nonresident family members was always relatively limited in Sweden, and would appear to have even increased its role in recent years rather than to have declined. In Israel, children living outside the elderly person's home also play a relatively small role in their support. The main impact of the greater availability of public support in present-day Sweden appears to be in reducing the roles of resident family, resident nonfamily, and friends and neighbors. In modern Israel, the group of those living alone is no greater proportionally than it was in Sweden in the 1950s, but it is the family that provides most of the care, whereas this has never been the case in Sweden.

CONCLUSION

We now summarize the implications of these findings in light of the questions raised at the outset of the paper. Firstly, we have seen that although the informal system may be more limited in an older and more advanced welfare state such as Sweden, it has by no means been eliminated there. Instrumental forms of informal support seem to be far more common than many of the observers of the Swedish scene would lead us to believe. Contacts and emotional support certainly remain widely prevalent. Secondly, at least in the case of Sweden, the more limited role of informal support seems to have preceded the period of major population aging and is related to longer-term cultural traditions with respect to institutionalization.

We have also found that differences between Israel and Sweden are very much related to differences in residential patterns. In both countries, elderly who live with their children are generally cared for by them without much external support. It is when the elderly live alone that the formal system has tended to replace the family. This pattern seems to be universal, characterizing both societies at all levels of development of formal support. The growth in formal support is related both to the rise in its use within the group of those not married and not living with children, and to the increase in the relative size of this group. This rise is related to the growth of separate residences made possible by the rise in living standards. At the same time, it has been facilitated by the increased availability of services.

However, most of the elderly do not live alone, residing for the most part with their spouse. This group has grown in the more advanced welfare societies over time. Thus, the overall balance of informal support is affected less by the process of population aging.

Finally, we consider the implications of our findings for the question of substitution between formal and informal support. It would appear that with the growth of formal support the extent of informal support has declined in Sweden in comparison to earlier periods. Similarly, the higher level of formal support in present-day Sweden, compared to Israel, is associated with a correspondingly lower level of informal support in Sweden. While informal support is still important, the findings suggest that at least some substitution occurs between formal and informal services.

Our findings are very relevant to the current debate in the United States, England and many other Western countries with respect to the future of informal support. They suggest that informal support will continue to play an important role in the care of the elderly. Therefore, policies need to be geared not only to developing alternatives, but also to strengthening the capacities of families to address this challenge. Attention needs to be given not only to children, however, but also to spouses, who are becoming more and more critical in fulfilling this role.

Moreover, our findings emphasize the importance of the extent of institutional services in determining the nature of the challenge faced by families in the community. If institutional services become less available and more and more elderly in need of personal care remain in the community, then co-residence with the family for at least some period may become more and more important. Similarly, home care services will need to shift their focus more and more to the direction of personal care.

AUTHOR NOTE

From 1982 to 1992, Jack Habib served as Director of the JDC-Brookdale Institute. He has published widely in the fields of gerontology, economics, and social welfare.

Gerdt Sundstrom is trained in sociology and social work, and has published and lectured widely in Sweden and abroad on old age care, family sociology, and related fields.

Karen Windmiller previously worked as a researcher at the JDC-Brookdale Institute in Israel.

REFERENCES

Andersson, L. (1985). An inquiry into preferred sources of support and help among a group of elderly Swedish women. Paper presented at the 13th International Congress of Gerontology, New York.

Be'er, S. & Factor, H. (1988). *Long-term care institutions and sheltered housing: The situation in 1987 and changes over time.* Jerusalem: JDC-Brookdale Institute of Gerontology, Jerusalem. (In Hebrew.)

Central Bureau of Statistics. (1962). *Demographic characteristics of the population, Part 1.* Publication No. 7. Jerusalem: State of Israel.

Central Bureau of Statistics. (1981). *1972 Census of population and housing: The aged in Israel.* Publication No. 17. Jerusalem: State of Israel.

Central Bureau of Statistics. (1986). *1983 Census of population and housing: The aged in Israel.* Publication No. 11. Jerusalem: State of Israel.

Central Bureau of Statistics. (1987a). *1987 Statistical abstracts of Israel*, No. 38. Jerusalem: State of Israel.

Central Bureau of Statistics. (1987b). *Labour force surveys 1985.* No. 801. Jerusalem: State of Israel.

Central Bureau of Statistics. (1988). *1985 Survey of persons aged 60 and over in households.* Jerusalem: State of Israel.

Christianson, J.B. (1988). The evaluation of the national long-term care demonstration: The effect of channeling on informal caregiving. *Health Services Research*, 23(1), 99-118.

Daatland, S. (1990). What are families for?: Or family solidarity and preference for help. *Ageing and Society*, 10(1),1-15.

Daatland, S. (1985). *Care of the aged in the Nordic countries: Trends and policies the last two decades.* Paper presented at the 13th International Congress of Gerontology, New York.

Factor, H., Guttman, M., & Shmueli, A. (1984). *Mapping of the long-term care system for the aged in Israel.* JDC-Brookdale Institute of Gerontology, Jerusalem.

Factor, H., Be'er, S., & Kaplan, I. (1986). *Mapping of community services for long-term care of the elderly in Jerusalem.* Jerusalem: JDC-Brookdale Institute of Gerontology.

Friis, H. (1977). The aged in Denmark, In I. Morton et al. (Eds.), *Reaching the aged: Social services in forty-four countries* (pp. 201-217). Beverly Hills, CA: Publications Inc.

Greene, V. (1983). Substitution between formally and informally provided care for the impaired elderly in the community. *Medical Care*, 21(6), 609-619.

Habib, J., & Cohen, M. (1990). Strategies for addressing the needs of the very old. *The social protection of the frail elderly* (pp. 177-205). International Social Security Association Studies and Research No. 28. Geneva.

Habib, J., & Windmiller, K. (1992). Family support to elderly persons in Israel. In H. Kendig, A. Hashimoto, & L. Coppard (Eds.), *Family support for the elderly: The international experience.* New York: Oxford University Press.

Habib, J., Factor, H., Naon, D., Brodsky, E., & Dolev, T. (1986). *Disabled elderly in the community: Developing adequate community-based services and their implications for the need for institutional placement.* Jerusalem: JDC-Brookdale Institute of Gerontology.

Habib, J., Sundstrom, G., & Windmiller, K. (In press). Understanding the differences in the patterns of support for elderly men and women: A comparison between Sweden and Israel.

Johnson, P., & Scott, P. (1988). *The economic consequences of population ageing in advanced societies.* Centre for Economic Policy Research Conference on Work, Retirement and Inter-generational Equity, 1850-2050.

Kemper, P., Applebaum, R., & Harrigan, M. (1987). Community care demonstrations: What have we learned? *Health Care Financing Review*, 8(4), pp. 87-100.

Lewis, M.A., Binstock, R., Cantor, M., & Schneewind, E. (1980). The extent to which informal and formal supports interact to maintain older people in the community. Paper presented at the 33rd Annual Meeting of the Gerontological Society of America, San Diego, California, November.

Morginstin, B. (1987). *Response of formal support systems to social changes and patterns of caring for the elderly.* Discussion Paper 36. Jerusalem: National Insurance Institute.

Morginstin, B. and Werner P. (1986). *Long-term care needs and provision of* services for the elderly: summary of selected data. Survey No. 51. Jerusalem: National Insurance Institute.

Noam, G., & Sicron, M. (1990). Socioeconomic trends among the elderly population in Israel: 1961-1983 analysis of census data. D-176-90. Jerusalem: JDC-Brookdale Institute of Gerontology.

Pinkerton, A., & Hill, D. (1984). Long-term care demonstration project of North San Diego County: Final report. San Diego: Allied Home Health Association.

Shmueli, A. (1989). Kinship networks in Israel. D-172-89. Jerusalem: JDC-Brookdale Institute of Gerontology.

Sjoberg, I. (1990). Personal communication.

Statistics Sweden. (1987). Statistical abstracts of Sweden.

Statistics Sweden. (1985a). 1976 Annual level-of-living survey. Report 18.

Statistics Sweden (1985b). Annual level-of-living survey, 1980-81. Report 43.

Statistics Sweden. (1977). 1975 Survey of elderly persons. Government White Paper. SOU. 9,100.

Statistics Sweden. (1956). 1954 Survey of elderly persons and survey of old age home clientele. Government White Paper 500:1.

Sundstrom, G. (1983). Caring for the aged in welfare society. Stockholm Studies in Social Work, No. 1 School of Social Work. Stockholm: University of Stockholm.

Sundstrom, G. (1984). How close? Distance and closeness in Swedish families. Mimeo. Stockholm: Riksforbund.

Sundstrom, G. (1985). Community care of the aged in Scandinavia. International Exchange Center on Gerontology.

Sundstrom, G. (1986). Family and state: Recent trends in the care of the aged in Sweden. Ageing and Society, 6,169-196.

Sundstrom, G. (1987). Old age care in Sweden. Stockholm: Swedish Institute.

Sundstrom, M. (1987). A study in the growth of part-time work in Sweden. Research Report No. 56. Stockholm: Arbetsliscentrum.

Torrey, B., Kinsella, K., & Taeuber, C. (1987). An aging world. International Population Reports. Series P-95. No. 78. U.S. Department of Commerce, Bureau of the Census. Washington, DC: U.S. Government Printing Office.

Tornstam, L. (1989). Formal and informal support for the elderly: An analysis of present patterns and future options in Sweden. Impact of Science on Society, No. 153, 39 (1), 57-64.

United Nations Demographic Yearbook. (1986). 38th Edition, Special Topic Natality Statistics.

Index